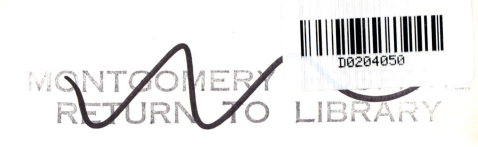

The Premenstrual Syndrome
and Progesterone Therapy

The Premenstrual Syndrome and Progesterone Therapy

Katharina Dalton FRCGP

Second Edition

WILLIAM HEINEMANN MEDICAL BOOKS LTD
London

YEAR BOOK MEDICAL PUBLISHERS INC
Chicago

First published 1977
by William Heinemann Medical Books Ltd
23 Bedford Square, London WC1B 3HH

Second Edition 1984

© Katharina Dalton, 1984

ISBN 0-433-07092-7 (UK)

Distributed in Continental North, South
and Central America, Puerto Rico,
Hawaii and the Philippines by
Year Book Medical Publishers Inc.

ISBN 0-8151-2266-7 (USA)

Year Book Code XK-2

Printed and bound in Great Britain at
The Camelot Press Ltd, Southampton

Contents

v

Preface
to the First Edition

In writing this book I have kept four clear aims in mind:

1. To bring within a small volume all that is known today about the premenstrual syndrome and its relationship to progesterone.
2. To clarify the differences between progesterone and progestogens and ensure a clear understanding of the basis for progesterone treatment. Also to provide full details of the treatment and management of those disorders which respond to progesterone.
3. To provide a practical handbook for the general practitioner, half of whose women patients are potential sufferers from the disease, and to enable physicians, psychiatrists, endocrinologists and others to recognise the syndrome when it occurs within their specialty and to understand its treatment. It is hoped that it will also be of value to social workers, health visitors and medical auxiliaries, enabling them to diagnose the syndrome and refer sufferers for treatment.
4. To provide a handy book reference for all who are concerned with the wellbeing of women. For this purpose each chapter is complete in itself, even though this incurs a certain amount of repetition and cross-reference.

References have been kept to a minimum, but for those who wish to go more fully into the subject or seek further enlightenment on any particular detail a list of the author's publications dealing specifically with the different aspects of the subject has been provided.

The somatic components of the premenstrual syndrome and

the value of progesterone in the treatment of premenstrual migraine were first recognised by Dr Raymond Greene, who also accepted clinical responsibility when I treated my first case of premenstrual asthma, epilepsy and rhinitis with progesterone. In those days we believed that the premenstrual syndrome was a rare condition, but we know now that it is the world's commonest, and probably the oldest, disease. Since those early days a considerable number of research workers have concentrated on the psychological aspects and hardly any attention has been given to the much more important somatic and hormonal aspects.

I take this opportunity of acknowledging how much Dr Raymond Greene has contributed to my understanding of this subject, and to thank him for all his guidance and encouragement. I have, indeed, been fortunate in having so many able people from professors to medical students who have contributed much by their criticism and stimulating discussions; particular mention must be made of Dr Christine Moore, Dr Gwyneth Sampson and Dr Sheila Handel who have all read the manuscript. My grateful thanks are extended to them all, especially my severest critics Dr Maureen Dalton and Dr Michael Dalton, and also to those most able typists Anita Dalton and Wendy Holton who have untiringly typed and retyped the manuscript and to Jean Mann who traced the hospital records. Finally, I must acknowledge my own indebtedness, and also that of all who read this book, to my husband, the Reverend Tom E. Dalton, and thank him for the many hours he has spent struggling with my nearly incomprehensible notes and often diffuse thoughts and translated them into very readable English.

Katharina Dalton
1977

Preface
to the Second Edition

A week is said to be a long time in politics; in the same way it is true that six years is a long time in medicine, because every minute someone, somewhere is discovering something new about human physiology, its ailments and foibles, their causes and treatments. So it is with premenstrual syndrome and progesterone therapy. The requirement of a new edition is a welcome opportunity to rewrite the whole book, incorporating the accumulated knowledge and experience of 35 years' intensive study and treatment of several thousands of PMS patients.

Today the public knows, or thinks it does, all about premenstrual syndrome, but this can never be so. In this edition my task has been to emphasise the precise *Definition* and *Diagnosis* and a full chapter has been allocated to each of these subjects. In view of the proliferation of much unprofitable reporting on premenstrual syndrome a new chapter has been included on *Clinical Studies* to bring to light the many difficulties and pitfalls of research into this subject, and the many hurdles the research worker has to negotiate to produce good scientific work.

The differences between natural progesterone and synthetic progestogens is still little understood by many medical specialists, who have difficulty anyway keeping up with the rapid advances in steroid chemistry, and particularly our understanding of progesterone receptors and the binding globulins. It gives me pleasure that it has fallen to the lot of my youngest daughter, Dr Maureen Dalton, to develop such a useful diagnostic test as the sex hormone binding globulin (SHBG) for the diagnosis of premenstrual syndrome. It has simplified my work and that of the many physicians whose energies are dedicated to the diagnosis and treatment of this syndrome. I am also grateful to my daughter Maureen for the chapters on *Aetiology* and *Progesterone and Progestogens*.

In writing this edition I have been aware of the needs of my American colleagues for an authoritative and informative book about premenstrual syndrome and progesterone responsive diseases.

Up-to-date statistical data on patients who have been treated by me with progesterone during 1982 are contained in the *Appendix*. My thanks go to Mrs Wendy Holton, Christine Fry, and Margaret Horne, Misses Janette Micklewright and Jane Rogers who extracted this data from my patients' records.

As with all my previous books and articles, this volume would never have reached fruition without the invaluable help of my husband and ghostwriter, the Reverend Tom Dalton, to whom I am most grateful. I am also indebted to Dr Sheila Handel, Dr Christine Moore, Dr Leslie Heard and Professor Louis Keith of Chicago for their invaluable criticism of the manuscript.

Katharina Dalton
1983

London W1

1

Introduction

Asthma, herpes, tonsillitis, acne, baby battering, epilepsy and alcoholic bouts may appear to have little in common. Nevertheless, in those cases in which there are regular recurrences during the premenstruum or menstruation, these symptoms all come within the classification of the premenstrual syndrome and will respond to progesterone therapy. The common factor in these apparently unrelated symptoms is their recurrence, always at the same time, in each menstrual cycle.

To appreciate why such a variety of symptoms should all respond to the same hormone, progesterone, we need only turn to Banting and Best's momentous discovery of insulin. Let us assume that their discovery had preceded Fehling's and Benedict's tests for the detection of glycosuria. Banting and Best would have found that insulin could cause a miraculous response in some cases of coma, a dramatic recovery in some cases of emaciation, perpetual fatigue and polyuria, and a marked improvement in some cases of carbuncles and peripheral neuritis. It was the use of Fehling's and Benedict's tests that enabled them to find a common factor in all these different symptoms, namely the presence of glycosuria. In the premenstrual syndrome there is a common factor: the cyclical recurrence of symptoms with each menstrual cycle. Unfortunately there is no single definitive test to assist the diagnosis of the premenstrual syndrome or, indeed, of progesterone deficiency, although there are hopeful signs on the horizon, and the estimation of the sex hormone binding globulin must be counted among them.

At present the recognition of this syndrome must depend upon the perception of the patient or of her doctor, and the confirmation of the cyclical recurrence on a menstrual chart.

It is now 35 years since progesterone was successfully used in the treatment of premenstrual syndrome. Today with a greater understanding of the hormonal basis of the disease, progesterone is still the specific treatment although the method of administration has been transformed as a result of the appreciation that progesterone is adequately absorbed by the rectal and vaginal routes.

Confusion among doctors regarding the differences between progesterone and progestogens led to incorrect treatment, and false conclusions were drawn from the failure of progestogens to relieve the somatic symptoms. Once the correct treatment has been started with the natural hormone progesterone, however, the results are quite dramatic. It is unfortunate that today only a minority of doctors in Great Britain and a handful of doctors in the United States are able and ready to diagnose premenstrual syndrome and treat it with progesterone. On the other hand, the general public, especially those who suffer from the syndrome, have a fuller understanding of the illness and its treatment than many of the doctors. It is essential, therefore, that an authoritative textbook should be available for the medical profession.

When progesterone was first isolated in 1932 its prime function was recognised as the proliferation of the endometrium and the maintenance of pregnancy (Allen). The profession used it eagerly for the treatment of severe pre-eclampsia, and of threatened or habitual abortion, albeit in inadequate doses and not selectively (Bennett, Marsden, McMann, Paterson, Young & Swyer). The fact that progesterone is species-specific is a stumbling block to the full understanding of the function of progesterone in menstruation and pregnancy. It should be mentioned here that pre-eclampsia is also species-specific and does not occur in other mammals. It is time for a reassessment of the part played by progesterone, not only in the disorders of menstruation, but also in the maintenance of pregnancy. This book goes part of the way towards such a reassessment but its main purpose is to ensure a full understanding of premenstrual syndrome and its treatment with progesterone.

2

Definition

The definition of premenstrual syndrome is 'the recurrence of symptoms in the premenstruum with absence of symptoms in the postmenstruum'.

It will be recognised that such a definition introduces a new concept into medical diagnosis. Medical diagnosis is usually dependent on the consideration of the type of symptoms, but in premenstrual syndrome, diagnosis is dependent on the timing of symptoms. Premenstrual syndrome covers an infinite variety of symptoms but the diagnosis can never be made solely on the basis of symptoms.

The first paper in British medical literature on the premenstrual syndrome was published in 1953 and was written jointly by Raymond Greene and myself. In it we recognised that the term 'premenstrual syndrome' was an imperfect description of the disease for, in this syndrome, the term 'premenstruum' is used loosely to cover the luteal phase of the menstrual cycle, that is from ovulation to menstruation. Definitively the premenstruum covers the four days immediately before menstruation; these are the days of greatest severity of symptoms in premenstrual syndrome, although symptoms may start at any time during the luteal phase. As the luteal phase never exceeds 16 days it is impossible for premenstrual symptoms to exceed 16 days. One must always be suspicious of the woman who claims that her premenstrual symptoms start on days eight or nine of her cycle; even in short cycles ovulation will rarely occur so early. Similarly, when a woman states that her premenstrual symptoms occur for a full three weeks before menstruation and then tries to explain the

3

long duration by claiming a cycle of five or more weeks, one must remain sceptical of her diagnosis.

Symptoms that have started during the premenstruum may continue during the first few days of menstruation. Occasionally symptoms start on the first or second day of scanty menstruation and before the onset of the full menstrual flow. Spotting in early menstruation is likely to occur in women fitted with an intra-uterine device.

Recurrence of symptoms means a repetition of symptoms for a minimum of three consecutive cycles. The severity of the symptoms may vary from one cycle to the next according to the degree of stress in the previous cycle; even so, the type of symptoms will remain basically the same. Thus one premenstruum may be characterised by headache and the following premenstruum by migraine with visual aura and prostration. Another woman may complain of premenstrual irritability characterised by shouting and screaming during some cycles and by actual physical violence during another cycle.

Absence of symptoms in the postmenstruum requires a phase of a minimum of seven days free from all symptoms. Most women experience two or three weeks without symptoms.

The term *premenstrual tension* covers only the psychological symptoms of tension, depression, irritability and lethargy. To use the term when the tension is overshadowed by more serious somatic symptoms, such as asthma, epilepsy or migraine, only confuses the diagnosis. The term premenstrual syndrome includes both the psychological and somatic symptoms.

When it was realised the recurring symptoms were at their peak during the last four days of the premenstruum and the first four days of menstruation, it became necessary to find a word to cover these vital eight days and the term *'paramenstruum'* was introduced to cover these two phases of the menstrual cycle. Various surveys have shown that in women about half of all such events as accidents, suicides, emergency hospital admissions and schoolgirls' punishments occur during the paramenstruum (Dalton) (Chapter 24).

In clinical studies the failure to adhere to the strict definition of premenstrual syndrome has resulted in confusion and consequently has produced conflicting results. This is also the probable explanation of the high rate of placebo response noted in controlled trials of drugs. Among the voluminous medical writings on the subject of premenstrual syndrome there are numerous examples of this failure: Reid and Yen (1981), for instance, did a review of premenstrual syndrome which contained over 300 references and produced 'a new hypothesis for the pathophysiology of PMS' and yet they failed to give any definition of premenstrual syndrome.

In *Behaviour and the Menstrual Cycle* (1982) edited by Friedman, five chapters are devoted to premenstrual tension, and reference to the subject occurs throughout the book. When the book was in its planning stage the author, who was invited to contribute a chapter on 'Premenstrual Tension: An Overview', emphasised to the editor the importance of using a common definition throughout the book and suggested a meeting or an exchange of correspondence with the other authors. The suggestion was rejected and now the reader is torn between using the author's strict criteria in one chapter and others using the term to cover tension and any other symptom that fluctuates with the menstrual cycle. Without a strict definition discussions on classification, aetiology and treatment lose their value. It is to overcome this difficulty that the definition of premenstrual syndrome is repeated at the beginning of the first ten chapters of this book.

Timing of symptoms
There are three common patterns of the timing of symptoms which come within the definition of premenstrual syndrome. The commonest pattern is that in which the symptoms occur for only a few days in the late premenstruum and then end suddenly with the onset of the full menstrual flow (Fig. 2.1 pattern A); the second pattern is that in which the symptoms start at ovulation, cease spontaneously within a day or two and then reappear during the last seven days of the premenstruum and finally disappear during menstruation (pattern B); the third pattern is found in those unfortunate women whose symptoms start abruptly at ovulation and gradually increase in severity throughout the entire luteal phase to cease during menstruation (pattern C). There are individual intermediate patterns in addition to the three common patterns shown but all of them occur within the luteal phase and merge imperceptibly. It should be noted that in all patterns the severity of symptoms is greatest during the last four premenstrual days. Although there are infinite variations of these patterns the

same type of pattern tends to recur in any one individual with each
menstrual cycle.

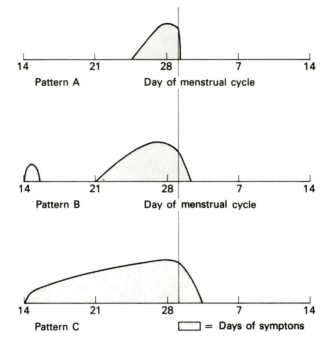

Fig. 2.1   Common patterns of timing of symptoms in premenstrual syndrome.

Menstrual distress

The commonest diagnostic error is to confuse premenstrual
syndrome with menstrual distress. Menstrual distress is defined
as: 'the presence of intermittent or continuous symptoms present
throughout the menstrual cycle which increase in severity during
the premenstruum or menstruation'.

This definition does not require that the recurrence of
symptoms always be at the same time in each menstrual cycle –
therefore, it can be diagnosed on the basis of only one cycle – nor
does it require the absence of symptoms in the premenstruum. It
should be appreciated that most chronic diseases have an
exacerbation of symptoms in relation to menstruation; one need
only cite depression, schizophrenia, migraine, rheumatoid
arthritis, chronic bronchitis, multiple sclerosis, tuberculosis and
glaucoma.

The timing of symptoms in menstrual distress also covers many variations; two examples are shown in Fig. 2.2 in which pattern D shows intermittent symptoms and pattern E shows continuous symptoms, but both have an exacerbation of symptoms in the paramenstruum.

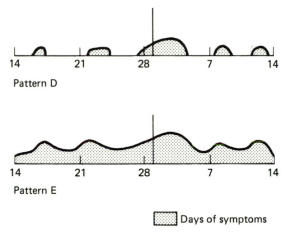

Pattern D

Pattern E

Days of symptoms

Fig. 2.2 Timing of symptoms of menstrual distress.

The menstrual cycle

To study the significance of the hormonal changes during the menstrual cycle it is important to divide it into phases of hormonal activity.

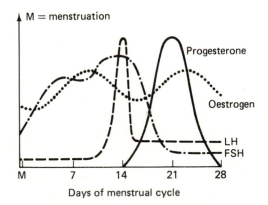

Days of menstrual cycle

Fig. 2.3 Menstrual hormone variations during the menstrual cycle. (From Dalton K. (1980) *Depression after Childbirth*. Fig 13, p 92.)

The conventional cycle of 28 days fits neatly into seven four-day phases having different levels of oestrogen and progesterone (Table 2). In adjusting for different lengths of cycles it is best to regard the luteal phase as being limited to 14 days and add to or subtract from the days of the late postmenstruum (days 9–12).

Table 2

Seven four-day phases of the menstrual cycle

Days	Phase	Oestrogen	Progesterone
1– 4	Menstruation	Low	Absent
5– 8	Early postmenstruum	Rising	Absent
9–12	Late postmenstruum	High	Absent
13–16	Ovulation	Falling	Low
17–20	Early luteal	Rising	Rising
21–24	Late luteal	High	High
25–28	Premenstruum	Falling	Falling

In some of the earlier work on the influence of menstruation, the menstrual cycle was arbitrarily divided into four phases of one week each (Gregory). This was a convenient division, but unfortunately it obscured the influence of the changing hormonal pattern with the result that during the premenstrual week the low incidence of events on days 22–24 was offset by the high incidence of events during days 25–28; likewise during the menstrual week the high incidence of events during days 1–4 was offset by the low incidence on days 5–7. The use of the seven-phase division clarifies the true hormonal picture.

The importance of using the seven phases of the menstrual cycle for studying the effect of the fluctuation of menstrual hormones is demonstrated in a survey into attempted suicide by Tonks and his colleagues. They divided the menstrual cycle into four weeks and found that 21 of 95 attempts were made during the menstrual week and 35 attempts during the premenstrual week. Thus 56 attempts were made during the menstrual and premenstrual weeks compared with an expected 47.5 attempts had there been an even distribution. When the menstrual cycle is divided into seven phases it is seen that 39 attempts were made during the paramenstruum compared with 27.1 attempts on an even distribution, a significant difference ($P = < 0.005$). In Fig. 2.4 Tonks's distribution of parasuicides is shown divided into four weeks, and below is the same distribution divided into the seven hormonal phases, a division which is used in most sociological studies.

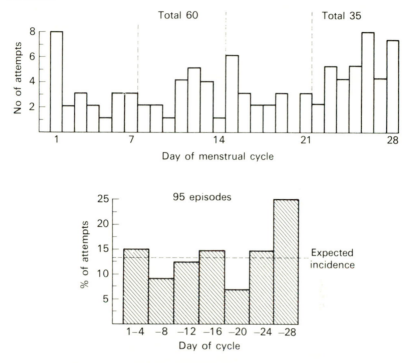

Fig. 2.4 Number of suicidal attempts in relation to the menstrual cycle. (From Tonks C.M., Rack P.H., Rose M.J. (1968). *J. Psychosom. Res.*; **2**:319.)

3

Diagnosis

Premenstrual syndrome is 'the recurrence of symptoms in the premenstruum with absence of symptoms in the postmenstruum'.

For the diagnosis this definition requires that:

1. Symptoms occur exclusively during the second half of the menstrual cycle.
2. Symptoms increase in severity as the cycle progresses.
3. Symptoms must be relieved by the onset of the full menstrual flow.
4. There must be an absence of symptoms in the postmenstruum.
5. Symptoms must have been present for at least three consecutive cycles.

A correct diagnosis depends on the accurate recording of symptoms day by day, together with a precise recording of the dates of menstruation. Nor should it be forgotten that the 28-day menstrual cycle is not the natural one, but is an average of all cycles, long and short. The artificial cycle produced by the contraceptive pill or other hormone preparations is precisely 28 days, but among women receiving no medication a cycle of 21–35 days is considered normal. A woman's cycle is considered regular if the length of the cycle does not vary by more than four days from cycle to cycle. There are very few women who can state precisely within one day the date of their next menstruation; it is far more usual for them to say – 'this coming weekend' or 'early next week'. There is only one positive method of diagnosis available today, and it is the best. It is the simple and inexpensive method of recording day by day the dates of the symptoms and the days of menstruation on a menstrual or frequency chart, such as is shown in Fig. 3.1. After 30 years' appreciation of premenstrual syndrome, one might have expected that by now the diary manufacturers would have included frequency charts in women's diaries.

The simplicity of recording encourages the cooperation of the patient. She is asked to mark with an 'M' in the appropriate square

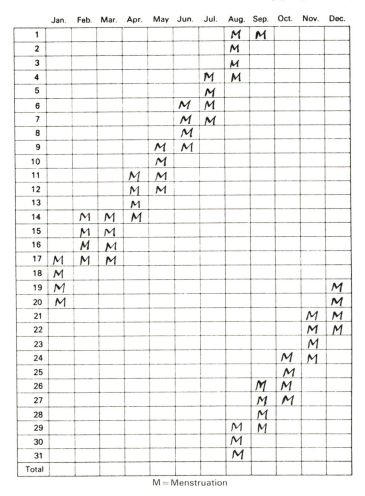

	Jan.	Feb.	Mar.	Apr.	May	Jun.	Jul.	Aug.	Sep.	Oct.	Nov.	Dec.
1								M	M			
2								M				
3								M				
4							M	M				
5							M					
6						M	M					
7						M	M					
8						M						
9					M	M						
10					M							
11				M	M							
12				M	M							
13				M								
14		M	M	M								
15		M	M									
16		M	M									
17	M	M	M									
18	M											
19	M											M
20	M											M
21											M	M
22											M	M
23											M	
24										M	M	
25										M		
26									M	M		
27									M	M		
28									M			
29								M	M			
30								M				
31								M				
Total												

M = Menstruation

Fig. 3.1   Chart showing 'perfect' cycle of 28 days and four days duration.

on the chart each day of her menstruation. If the menstrual bleeding is slight or scanty she should use a small 'm'. If the 'M's on the chart group along a horizontal line the length of the menstrual cycle is 30–31 days, allowing for the varying lengths of the calendar months. If the line of 'M's runs obliquely upwards the cycle length is shorter and if the 'M's slant downwards the cycle length is longer than the calendar month (Fig. 3.2).

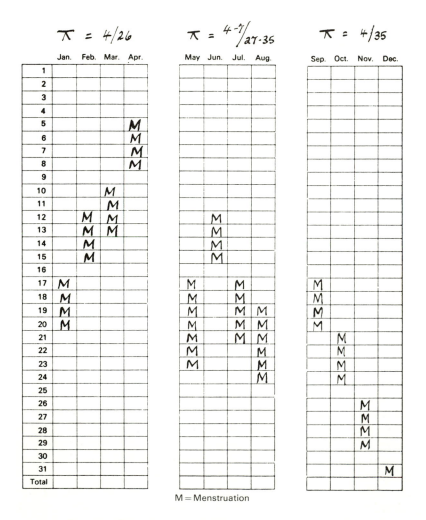

Fig. 3.2 Chart showing variations in the menstrual cycle.

The calendar in Fig. 3.3, in which the days of menstruation are marked, is shown for comparison. It is difficult at a glance to decide whether there is a regular or irregular cycle or if it is a long or a short cycle. The difficulty in interpreting the data from a calendar is increased when the dates on which symptoms occur have been added. The only advantage of a calendar is to show at a glance when symptoms always occur on the same day of the week, irrespective of menstruation, but this would have nothing to do with premenstrual syndrome.

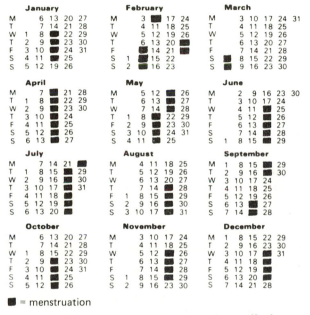

■ = menstruation

Fig. 3.3 Calendar with menstruation marked.

Various designs for menstrual charts are in use and it may seem immaterial whether it is drawn vertically or horizontally, but it is easier if a whole year's menstruations can be seen at a glance, rather than having to follow the line across two or more pages. The vertical chart avoids this complication but keeps the chart compact. Some charts suggest starting the recording on the first day of each menstrual cycle, rather than the beginning of the calendar month. This has the disadvantage that with varying lengths of cycle it is not always easy to determine the duration of symptoms, whether they continue until menstruation or stop for a day or two before menstruation.

Some charts have been designed only for women with cycles of 31 days, neglecting those with longer cycles. Others are designed to cover one month only and ask specifically about certain symptoms. An example of such a poor design is shown in Fig. 3.4 which does not inquire about the length of menstruation, it is useless for women with long cycles, and combines two distinctly separate symptoms of 'headache and depression' in one column.

Although the design of the chart may seem immaterial, on reflection the importance of a standard design becomes evident. When a busy doctor is seeing ten women, each of whom has a chart of a different design, much of his time will be taken up in sorting out the data that have been presented in so many different ways. When the charts are of a standard design it is possible at a glance to interpret accurately each patient's individual pattern of menstruation and the relationship of the symptoms shown. The importance of having a whole year's menstrual pattern available on one small card can never be overemphasised. The chart in Fig. 3.1 has been in use for over 35 years; the test of long usage has shown that it is simple to use and easily covers all the requirements. A supply can be obtained from *Drug and Therapeutics Bulletin*, Consumers' Association, 14 Buckingham Street, London WC2.

The patient is asked to mark on the chart, with an appropriate symbol, the days on which menstruation occurs and the days when symptoms are present. The symbols are chosen individually for each woman and might include 'B' for breast tenderness, 'H' for headache, 'X' for pain. Capital letters 'B', 'H', 'X', may be used as symbols for severe symptoms and small letters 'b', 'h', 'x' for mild symptoms but no more than three symbols should be used for each patient, and these should be the three priority presenting symptoms. Some symptoms are easier to chart than others. For instance, a headache usually has a definite beginning and end, whereas with tiredness the beginning might be imperceptible (Fig. 3.5).

In premenstrual syndrome the symptoms may group around the time of menstruation with the postmenstrual days free from symptoms. Ovulatory attacks stand out clearly on the chart (Fig. 3.6).

These charts may be given to the husband or mother to record at

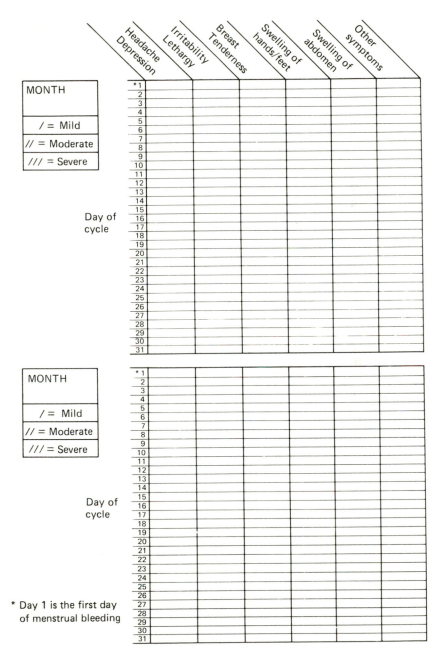

Fig. 3.4 Unhelpful menstrual chart.

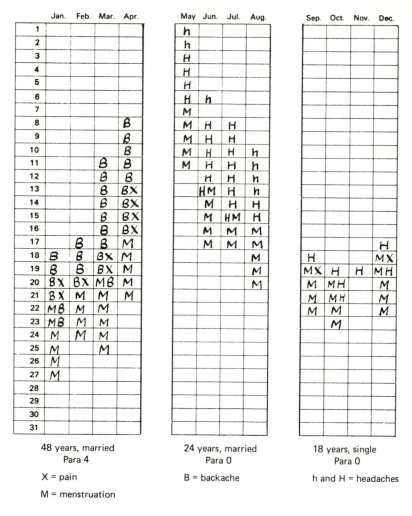

48 years, married
Para 4

24 years, married
Para 0

18 years, single
Para 0

X = pain   B = backache   h and H = headaches

M = menstruation

Fig. 3.5   Typical charts of sufferers from premenstrual syndrome.

the same time as the patient, they can then record the days when they feel that she is being unreasonable or seems to be unduly depressed. The charts may be used for children with recurrent symptoms such as colds, enuresis, temper tantrums and so on, and then superimposed on the mother's chart to determine if there is any correlation (see Chapter 25). The charts are also useful in charting premenarcheal girls, postmenopausal women and

	Jan.	Feb.	March	April
1				X
2				X
3				X
4				X
5		X		X
6		X	X	M X
7		X	X	M
8		X	X	M
9		X	X	M
10		X	M	
11	X	M X	M	
12	X	M	M	
13	X	M		
14	M	M		
15	M			
16	M			
17				
18				
19				
20				
21				X
22				
23			X	
24				
25				
26				
27		X		
28	X			
29				
30				
31				

X = attack of symptoms

M = menstruation

Fig. 3.6 Chart showing premenstrual syndrome with attacks at ovulation.

those who have had a hysterectomy. Their cyclical pattern will still show up and the symptoms will respond to treatment. At the menopause the chart may show that headaches, vertigo, backache and other symptoms still occur at the times of missed menstruation. Menstruation after a prolonged gap tends to occur about the times of expected menstruation, as forecast by continuing the line of 'M's across the chart (Fig. 3.7).

	Jan.	Feb.	March	April	May	June	July	Aug.	Sept.	Oct.	Nov.	Dec.
1												
2												
3												
4												
5												
6												
7												
8												
9												
10												
11												
12	X									X		
13	X									X		
14	X								X	X	X	
15	M	X						X	X	X	X	
16	M	X	X	X			X	X	M	X	X	X
17	M	X	X	X			X	M	M		X	X
18		X	M	X	X		X	M	M			X
19		M	M	X	X	X	X	M				X
20		M	M	X	MX	X						
21		M			M							
22					M							
23												
24												
25												
26												
27												
28												
29												
30												
31												

X = symptoms

M = menstruation

Fig. 3.7 Cyclical symptoms continuing at the menopause.

If, in women who are amenorrhoic, symptoms are shown to be occurring cyclically, the response to treatment is likely to be as good as if menstruation was accompanying the symptoms.

Symptoms limited to the postmenstruum are extremely rare and any patient claiming such a relationship of symptoms to menstruation should be asked to keep a careful record for a few months before accepting such a claim. Symptoms occurring after the periods may be ovulatory attacks – that is, they occur a week after the end of menstruation.

Before treatment it is essential to obtain a good record of the individual's normal duration of bleeding and length of cycle. Hormones may either lengthen or shorten the cycle or the duration of the bleed and without knowledge of the patient's norm it is difficult to distinguish any alteration in an individual patient which can be attributed to the treatment. The difference between the characteristics of the cycle that the patient claimed at her initial interview and those of the menstrual pattern shown later on her menstrual chart is often remarkable. Most women incorrectly claim to have a regular menstrual cycle of 28 days, this idea reflecting what they were taught to expect in biology lessons at school.

Charts from women suffering from menstrual distress can easily be recognised at a glance for their symptoms occur irregularly throughout the month, and in particular there are symptoms in the postmenstruum (Fig. 3.8).

Chronic diseases are usually exacerbated at times of menstruation – for example, rheumatoid arthritis, Crohn's disease, pyrexia in tuberculosis and oedema in cardiac disease – and patients may allay fears that their general condition is deteriorating by charting the days of exacerbation.

Not all women who have episodic symptoms have them in relation to menstruation; there may be other unrecognised precipitating factors such as food, stress or allergies occurring on one particular day of the week, or at weekends or holidays. If this is suspected the information on the chart may be transposed to the day of the week (Fig. 3.9).

The chart in Fig. 3.9 was from a 27-year-old secretary, who had migraine attacks at fortnightly intervals, originally on Tuesdays but later on Thursdays. It was only by keeping a careful record that it became obvious that these migraine attacks were unrelated to menstruation, which occurred at an interval of 29–30 days. Further questioning as to what Tuesday activity had been transferred to Thursday, showed that on Tuesday she went direct to the hairdresser from work having had only a snack lunch. The migraine developed on her way home at about 2000 hours. When her favourite hairdresser changed her late night to Thursdays the patient changed her appointment to that day. In her case

Day	Jan.	Feb.	March	April	May	June	July	Aug.	Sept.	Oct.	Nov.	Dec.
1			M					X		X		
2						X	X					
3				X								
4			X									
5										X	X	
6	M				X							
7	M	X							X			X
8	M	X	X						X			
9	M		X	X			X		X			
10	X						X		X			
11	X			MX						X		X
12				M		M				X		X
13			X	M	M	M	X	M		X		
14		X		X	MX	M	MX	MX	X		X	
15				X	M	M	M	M	M			
16					M		M	M	M			
17	X	X						M	M	XM		
18		X	X				X	M	M		M	M
19			M		X			M	M		M	M
20			M	X				X			M	M
21	X		M							MX		M
22	X	X	M						X	M		
23								X	X	M	X	
24		X							X	M	X	
25		X	X		X		X			X	X	X
26		X	X							X		
27	X	M	X									
28	X	M				X						
29	MX			X					X			
30	M		X						X	X		
31	M									X		X

Fig. 3.8   Charts of women with menstrual distress.

the migraine attacks were due to fasting and not related to menstruation (Dalton, 1973).

Another example was seen in a Cypriot housewife with an unmanageable child. She was referred with numerous psychosomatic symptoms, including abdominal pains, possibly at mid-cycle. When she returned after a month it was possible after

Sunday   –
Monday   –
Tuesday   1111
Wednesday   –
Thursday   111111
Friday   –
Saturday   –

	Jan.	Feb.	Mar.	Apr.	May	Jun.	Jul.	Aug.	Sep.	Oct.	Nov.	Dec.
1						H						
2												
3												
4												
5												
6												
7												
8										H		
9									H			
10												
11												
12							H					
13							H					
14												
15						H						
16												
17												
18												
19						M						
20						M	M					
21						M	M	M				
22							M	M				
23							MH					
24												
25												
26												
27							H					
28												
29						H	H					
30												
31												
Total												

H = migraine   M = menstruation

Fig. 3.9   Chart showing attacks at fortnightly intervals. (From Dalton K. (1973) *J. Roy. Coll. Gen. Pract.)*

examining the chart to guess that her husband worked late on Saturday, but had his half-day on Thursday. Pains were absent when father was at home to accept responsibility for the naughty boy on Thursday and Sunday, but pains increased in severity when the mother had to cope alone with the child all day on Saturday and put him to bed.

Monthly attacks of symptoms unrelated to menstruation may be noted among those in stockbrokers, accountancy and wages offices where the stress of work at the end of each month may precipitate symptoms. In other cases a monthly social or even the husband's monthly sales conference may be the root cause.

The fact that symptoms always occur on one day of the week are not always quite so easily explained. An adopted 16-year-old girl had asthmatic attacks on Monday, not every week but always on that day. The psychiatrist explained this by the patient being at home at weekends and being reminded of her adoption. The allergist's explanation was her allergy to house dust, for at weekends she would clean her room. A three-month calendar revealed that she had an unusually precise menstrual cycle of 28 days, although she was not on oral contraceptives, and attacks were occurring on the 28th day and occasionally on the 14th day; her menstruation started on Tuesdays. She responded to progesterone therapy.

Patients can often help with past dates by searching the pages of their diaries and producing definite evidence of the dates of previous attacks and of menstruation; these are easily recalled if they coincide with an important event like Christmas, weddings and holidays. On one occasion when the author was trying to arrange a social gathering, the secretary of the society produced her diary to see if a proposed date was suitable. 'No', she declared, 'I'll be having a migraine attack on that day.' Some patients make a note of forthcoming attacks.

Biochemical assays

The only useful diagnostic biochemical test for premenstrual syndrome is sex hormone binding globulin binding capacity (SHBG) estimated by Iqbal and Johnson's two-tier method (see Chapter 9). In 50 well-diagnosed severe cases of premenstrual syndrome it was shown to be below 50 nmol DHT/litre compared with 50 controls who were at the normal female level of 50–80 nmol/litre (Dalton M., 1981) (Fig. 3.10). However, the SHBG must

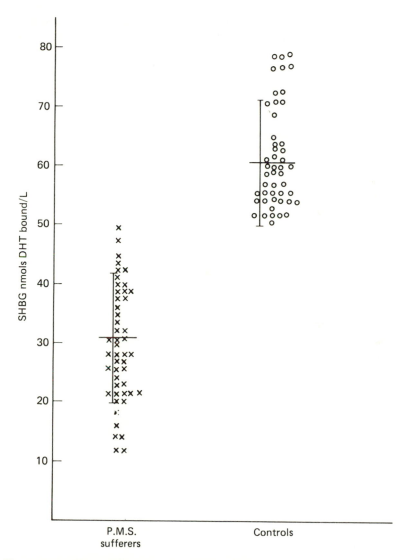

Fig. 3.10 SHBG-binding capacity in 50 patients with severe premenstrual syndrome compared with 50 controls.

be tested while women are free from all medication, including the pill, sedatives and simple analgesics. Altered SHBG levels also occur in obese women, those with thyroid disease, hirsutism and in some women in the ethnically hirsute races.

While there is much to support the hypothesis that progesterone deficiency, either absolute or relative, plays a part in the aetiology of premenstrual syndrome, there is as yet little evidence that the costly isolated radioimmunoassays of total progesterone levels during the premenstruum are helpful. Progesterone is secreted episodically in 20-minute spurts, so single blood samples are of only limited value in assessing the competence of the hypothalamic-pituitary-ovarian pathways. Furthermore, serum progesterone is mostly bound and it is the free fraction of progesterone that is of significance. Tests of salivary progesterone are being developed and these may prove to be valuable because the salivary progesterone is considered to be free and unbound.

Measures of serum progesterone level, when tested seven days before menstruation, are valuable in determining if ovulation has occurred, but they are of no value in diagnosing premenstrual syndrome because premenstrual syndrome can also occur in an anovular cycle. The 24-hour collection of urine for estimating pregnandiol, the major metabolite of progesterone, is unreliable although urine is the main pathway for the excretion of progesterone metabolites; a variable proportion is also excreted via the bile, faeces, expired air and the skin.

Basal temperature chart

Deficiency of progesterone may be shown up on a basal temperature chart where the normal rise occurs at ovulation, but then the temperature falls showing a deficient luteal phase. It has been estimated that among a group of apparently normal women 5% show anovular cycles and 12.5% a defective luteal phase (Fig. 3.11).

A normal menstrual cycle has been defined as one showing all the following features:

1. Mid-cycle peak of luteinising hormone.
2. Luteal phase lasting 12–16 days.
3. Progesterone values greater than 5 ng/ml 5–8 days after the surge of luteinising hormone.

Giving progesterone during the second half of the cycle produces a raised basal temperature. Nevertheless, it should be emphasised that premenstrual syndrome does not depend on ovulation – indeed it can occur at times of missed menstruation, at the menopause and after oophorectomy.

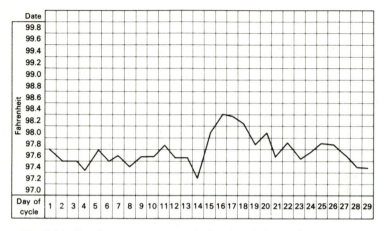

Fig. 3.11 Basal temperature graph showing defective luteal phase.

Attack forms

Some of the acute episodes which may occur in this syndrome appear to result from relative hypoglycaemia, common during the premenstruum. If this is suspected the use of an attack form as in Fig. 3.12 provides valuable information (Dalton, 1973).

Name..   Date ....
                Day of week ....
                Time of onset...
                Duration..
Day of cycle..   Days before next menstruation............................

During the 24 hours *before* the attack:—

(1) Did you have any special worry, overwork or shock?

(2) What had you done during the day?
        Normal work?
        Unusual activity?
        Extra tired?

(3) What food had you eaten and when?

        Breakfast ....   Time...
....
        Mid-morning.......................................   Time...
....
        Lunch ....   Time...
....
        Mid-afternoon.....................................   Time...
....
        Supper ....   Time...
....
        Evening...   Time...
....
        Bedtime ....   Time...
....

Fig. 3.12 Attack form. (From Dalton K. (1973). *J. Roy. Coll. Gen. Pract.*)

It may be used in cases of migraine, fainting, aggressive outbursts, phobic panic attacks, epileptic fits and any symptoms with an acute onset that can be accurately timed. The patient is asked to complete an attack form immediately after each of her next three attacks, stating all that she has done, and particularly all the food she has consumed, during the 24 hours immediately preceding the attack. The forms give quick and accurate information which if sought several days later would take much more time and would not provide the accurate information required. The questions are so phrased that they cover women who have a short cycle of 21 days or a long one of 35 days.

It is surprising how frequently one meets women with acute premenstrual attacks which occur after long intervals without food. A 22-year-old part-time teacher was referred by a psychiatrist for premenstrual weeping attacks which occurred 'at all times of the day and apparently without provocation'. The menstrual chart confirmed that they were occurring during the late prementruum, while the attack form showed that the attacks were preceded by several hours of fasting. The patient had noticed that she always gained weight premenstrually and so she dieted stringently at this time. When seen at 1700 hours she had been weeping spontaneously in the waiting room, and later stated that she had had only a small helping of cereals for breakfast at 0800 hours and an apple for lunch as she was going out to dinner with friends later. Avoiding fasting cured the weeping.

Menstrual distress questionnaires

The Moos menstrual distress questionnaire (MMDQ) is a useful tool for diagnosing menstrual distress, for which it was devised, but it is of no value in diagnosing premenstrual syndrome (Moos, 1968 & 1969).

The diagnosis of menstrual distress depends on the day by day variations in mood and severity of symptoms in relation to menstruation but, unlike premenstrual syndrome, it does not require a symptom-free phase in the postmenstruum. It is a psychologically orientated questionnaire, excluding somatic symptoms, and asks the woman to rate on a six-point scale the severity of some 47 symptoms, the severity scale ranging from 'no experience' to 'disturbing experience'. Moos differentiated eight symptom clusters in the questionnaire in the areas of pain, concentration, behaviour change, automatic reactions, water retention, affect, arousal and control. The pain clusters include muscle stiffness, headaches, cramps, backache, fatigue and general aches and pains, so the questionnaire does not relate specifically to the premenstrual syndrome, but can also include the pain symptoms of spasmodic dysmenorrhoea or endometriosis. Sampson and Jenner (1977) have described a method of analysing the data from the questionnaires using sine waves to assess quantitatively the complaints associated with menstruation, but this also fails to differentiate premenstrual syndrome from menstrual distress because it cannot single out that essential feature of diagnosis – an absence of symptoms in the postmenstruum. Sampson in her paper, 'Premenstrual Syndrome – Double Blind Controlled Trial of Progesterone and Placebo' (1979), used the Moos menstrual distress questionnaire in the study. She included a figure in the paper which showed the presence of symptoms in the postmenstruum in the first and second cycle before treatment started. In a subsequent issue of the *British Journal of Psychiatry* it was suggested that the article should have been entitled 'Menstrual Distress – a Double Blind Controlled Trial of Progesterone and Placebo' (Dalton, 1980).

The use of questionnaires for studying symptoms in the menstrual cycle has been questioned by Parlee, Zimmerman and others on statistical grounds. They suggested that the studies may be supporting cultural stereotypes rather than actual valid scientific findings and there was a failure to assess the stability of the scores and the test-retest reliability. In fact, when the original questionnaire was designed, nearly half of the subjects were taking oral contraceptives, over half had not yet had children, 10% were pregnant and 5% did not reply to the question concerning the use of contraception. Such a population is inappropriately diverse.

Furthermore, the Moos menstrual distress questionnaire cannot be used by those with a poor command of the English language who may not be able to recognise the difference between 'distractable' and 'difficulty in concentration' or between 'decreased efficiency' and 'lowered school or work performance'. Moreover how many people could assess on a six-point scale 'lowered motor coordination', even if they knew what it meant?

Another method sometimes used in the diagnosis of menstrual distress is by day-to-day assessment of mood using the visual analogue scales. Women are asked to mark on a 100mm lineal scale their appropriate mood for the day in terms of depression, sadness, tension, bloatedness, loss of libido, aggression, lethargy and anxiety. The score is measured by the distance of their mood mark along the line and a total score for the day is then obtained. The difference in value between the preovulatory and pre-menstrual score gives the Premenstrual Mood Index (PMI). It should be appreciated that whereas a decrease in libido is calculated as a positive symptom of menstrual distress, in premenstrual syndrome many women experience an increase in libido in the premenstruum (Aitken).

There is no relationship between the severity and duration of symptoms present in premenstrual syndrome. The explosion of symptoms which may occur in cases of epilepsy, baby battering and drug overdose may last only an hour and need not be accompanied by bloatedness, breast tenderness or alteration in libido, and thus would merit a low score in the Moos menstrual distress questionnaire or the visual analogue scale. Furthermore, the introspection required for the conscientious completion of the 47 items on the Moos menstrual distress questionnaire daily for a minimum of two months, demands highly motivated individuals, such as might be either neurotic or obsessional.

Retrospective diagnosis

In criminal cases it is particularly helpful to be able to obtain accurate retrospective information to confirm the diagnosis of premenstrual syndrome. While some women can consult their diaries and give dates of menstruation and dates of previous severe symptoms, in other cases the necessary information has to be found by perusing prison documents, police records, work or school absences or school punishment books.

As example of a retrospective search requiring the scrutiny of such sources of information was in respect of an 18-year-old student charged with arson (Dalton, 1980). She had been of exemplary behaviour until her menarche at 13 years, but by the age of 14 she was having episodes of bizarre behaviour which the parents could not understand. On one occasion she set fire to her bedroom curtains. After an interval she ran away from home and was returned by the police, then unexpectedly she shaved her head and her eyebrows; a few weeks later she slashed her fingers and sought help from the local hospital. The precise dates were obtained by finding the date of the insurance claim, information from the local police, the date of the cheque when the parents bought her a wig to cover her shaven head and the date the casualty officer sutured her fingers. These events occurred at intervals of 28–32 days, although the precise dates of menstruation were unknown. It was two years later that she committed arson and was taken to prison immediately and the records show that she was menstruating at the time. Within a few days she was released on bail, but exactly one month later she was charged with being drunk and disorderly while on bail. She was returned to prison and again it was noted that she was menstruating. She was again released on bail, but a month later she took an overdose and had a short hospital admission, her hospital notes revealing that she was menstruating. After three months there was another more serious case of arson at her father's house. She was committed to prison and noted to be menstruating. The following month while still in prison she slashed her wrists and the next day tried to strangle herself by fixing a sheet to the top of the window. She was again noted to be menstruating. This retrospective information was used to confirm the diagnosis of premenstrual syndrome. She received progesterone treatment, experienced normal menstruations and was released on probation. Now three years later she is leading a normal happy life with a successful career.

Another example of retrospective scrutiny which confirmed the diagnosis of premenstrual syndrome occurred in the case of a 28-year-old worker in the food industry, who was accused of fatally stabbing her girl friend. Following the stabbing she was admitted to prison and noted to be menstruating. Her menarche had been at the age of 15 years, and since the age of 16 she had received 26 convictions for offences varying from causing criminal damage, assault, theft, trespassing, writing threatening letters, possessing dangerous weapons and, finally, to murder. A psychiatrist described her in the prison documents as 'most of the time she is pleasant and cooperative, but at times she loses her senses and can be quite impulsive'. Recorded in her prison documents were 30 separate episodes of impulsive bizarre behaviour, which included trying to set fire to the bed in her cell, trying to escape, strangling, attempted drowning, smashing windows, cutting her wrists and assault. The precise dates of these eposides of violence in prison and of her previous offences were noted. Then with the assistance of a statistician, an analysis of the dates revealed that an average cycle length of 29.55 ± 1.45 days could be fitted in between episodes of violence while in prison (Fig. 3.12) and an average cycle length of 29.04 days ± 1.47 days could be fitted in between the prison admissions (Fig. 3.14). The judge accepted this evidence of premenstrual syndrome, she was treated for five months with progesterone while she was in prison and, as there had been no further episodes of distressed behaviour in prison, she was released on probation.

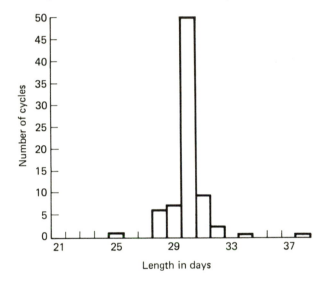

Fig. 3.13   Distribution of 'fitted' cycles between episodes of violence in prison. (*Lancet* (1980) 1080.)

Diagnostic pointers

The diagnosis of premenstrual syndrome depends entirely on the correlation of symptoms during the premenstruum and the absence of symptoms in the postmenstruum. Even so, there are some useful diagnostic pointers which can be obtained at the initial interview and can indicate the women who are most at risk.

Time of onset and increased severity

Premenstrual syndrome tends to start and also to increase in severity at those times in a woman's life when marked changes in hormone levels are occurring, such as take place at puberty, following a pregnancy, during or after taking oral contraceptives,

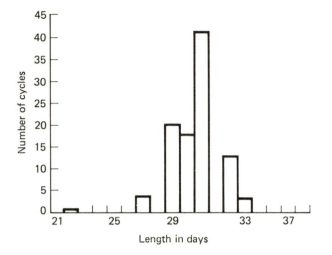

Fig. 3.14 Distribution of 'fitted' cycles between prison admissions. (Dalton K. *Lancet* (1980) 1081.)

after a period of amenorrhoea and following sterilisation. The frequency of a hormonal event being regarded by the patient as the starting time of premenstrual syndrome is shown in Table 3.1, and as the time of increased severity in Table 3.2 (see Appendix Table 27.6 & 27.7).

Table 3.1

Time of onset of premenstrual syndrome

(Patients first seen in 1981 and 1982 n=236)		
	n	%
Puberty	66	28
After pregnancy	67	28
Postnatal depression	22	8
Pill	10	4
Hysterectomy/oophorectomy	6	2
Sterilisation	5	2
Amenorrhoea	4	2
Hormonal event	180	76
Non-hormonal event	29	12
Unknown	27	12

Table 3.2

Time of increased severity of premenstrual syndrome

	n=58 n	%
After pregnancy	33	58
Pill	9	15
Postnatal depression	5	9
Amenorrhoea	4	7
Sterilisation	3	5
Hysterectomy/oopherectomy	1	1
Hormonal event	55	95
Non-hormonal event	3	5

The results of recent studies support the possibility that plasma concentration of progesterone may be reduced in patients who have had bilateral tubal ligations (Radwanska *et al.* 1979).

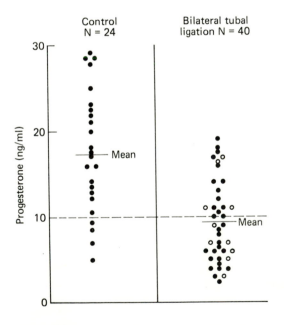

Fig. 3.15　Progesterone levels after bilateral tubal ligation. (After Radwanska E. *et al.* (1978). *Obstet. Gynecol.*; **54**:789–792.)

Painless menstruation

Painless menstruation is a characteristic of premenstrual syndrome. Indeed the very reason why many sufferers of migraine, epilepsy and asthma fail to recognise the time relationship of attacks is that menstruation is so uneventful that the timing of its comings and goings pass unnoticed. Spasmodic dysmenorrhoea, in the form of severe cramping pains in the lower abdomen, possibly radiating down the inner side of the thighs, coinciding with the onset of menstruation and increasing in intensity on the first day of menstruation, rarely occurs in premenstrual syndrome. Heaviness and dragging of the lower abdomen may be present some days before menstruation, being relieved by the full menstrual flow (Chapter 19).

Increase in libido during the premenstruum

Israel was the first in 1938 to draw attention to the increase in libido in the premenstruum among sufferers of premenstrual syndrome and it has been confirmed by Grey, Hart, Corner and Shader *et al.* It is this increase in libido which distinguishes premenstrual syndrome from a depressive illness in which there is a decrease in libido throughout the cycle.

Inability to tolerate the oral contraceptives

Women with premenstrual syndrome have difficulty in tolerating oral contraceptives, and are the ones who change brands and finally stop this method because of depression, headaches, weight gain and an increase in their premenstrual symptoms. This is in distinct contrast to those suffering from spasmodic dysmenorrhoea who experience good symptomatic relief, those with menorrhagia who benefit from the lighter menstruation and those with irregular menstruation who appreciate the reliability of regular menstruation. This intolerance was emphasised in the survey in 1982 of 290 new patients, who had used oral contraceptives (Table 3.3), and is further seen in Tables 27.8 & 27.9 in the Appendix. Some of these women, who experienced no side effects on the pill, used oral contraceptives before the pregnancy which resulted in the start of their premenstrual syndrome.

Weight fluctuations

Premenstrual syndrome women experience monthly swings of 3–4kg and, in adult life, swings exceeding 12kg are common.

Table 3.3

Effect of pill

	n=290	
	n	%
No side effects	60	12
Side effects, stopped the pill	230	89

Reported side effects

	n=230	
	n	%
Depression	60	26
Headache	58	25
Weight gain	31	13
Increased PMS	26	11
Nausea	18	8
Bloatedness	12	5
Loss of libido	11	5
Breast tenderness	10	4
Tiredness	10	4

Comparison of the highest-ever weight, excluding pregnancy, with the lowest-ever weight since the teenage years should be included in the medical history. It is irrelevant whether at the time of interview she is at her highest-ever or lowest-ever weight.

Altered hunger tolerance during the menstrual cycle

Sufferers from premenstrual tension cannot tolerate long intervals without food, and complain that their lives consist of episodes of dieting and strict fasting during the postmenstruum followed by uncontrolled cravings and binges during the premenstruum (Smith & Saunder). The onset of acute symptoms (violence, panic attacks and migraine) often occur after long gaps between eating, exceeding 5 hours by day or 13 hours overnight. Attack forms may be used to investigate the food gaps.

Altered tolerance to alcohol during the menstrual cycle

The patient may find that whereas she can tolerate a definite amount of her favourite drink on most days, during the premenstruum she becomes intoxicated on less than her usual amount. There may also be urges to drink alcohol in the premenstruum which are absent at other times of the cycle.

Effect of pregnancy

Sufferers usually conceive easily but most of them experience an exceptionally severe and prolonged attack of symptoms at the time of their first menstruation. They are liable to have a threatened abortion in the first trimester, but then most of them go on to be exceptionally well in pregnancy and free from their usual premenstrual symptoms (especially migraine, asthma and epilepsy). Those few whose symptoms continue throughout pregnancy are likely to develop pre-eclampsia. The incidence of premenstrual syndrome after pre-eclampsia is high, 78% after one pregnancy, rising to 100% after four pregnancies (Dalton, 1954). Postnatal depression, severe enough to require medical attention, frequently heralds the onset of premenstrual syndrome (Dalton, 1980). The survey reported in the appendix revealed that of 769 women, who had experienced a full-term pregnancy, as many as 59% had subsequently suffered from postnatal depression. This high incidence of postnatal depression among women with premenstrual syndrome suggests the possibility of a common aetiological factor. It also emphasises the need for pregnant women who are known to suffer from premenstrual syndrome to be offered prophylactic progesterone therapy against postnatal depression (Dalton, 1980) (Chapter 21). (See Appendix Table 27.11).

Diagnostic checklist

When a reliable two-month menstrual calendar is not immediately available or is ambiguous a checklist such as shown in Table 3.4 is useful in recognising high-risk individuals, but it is not a positive diagnosis. Items are scored 'not relevant', 'positive' or 'negative'. Items which might be marked 'non-relevant' would include the effect of the pill in a non-user, the complications of pregnancy in a nulliparous woman, and the altered tolerance to hunger or alcohol in those who have not previously considered this possibility. Women presenting with spasmodic dysmenorrhoea score two negatives and women who have had pregnancies uncomplicated by threatened abortion, pre-eclampsia or postnatal depression score one negative for each normal pregnancy. The total positive scores are multiplied by 100 and divided by the sum of positive and negative scores to give a percentage. Women complaining of premenstrual symptoms who present with a diagnostic check list of over 66% are the most likely to produce a positive menstrual calendar at a later date (Dalton, 1982).

Table 3.4

Diagnostic checklist

	Not relevant	Positive	Negative
Time of onset (puberty, pill, pregnancy, amenorrhoea)			
Time of increased severity (pill, pregnancy, amenorrhoea and sterilisation)			
Painless menstruation (Score 2 negatives if period pain is presenting symptom)			
Increased libido in premenstruum			
Threatened abortion			
Pre-eclampsia			
Postnatal depression			
Side effects with oral contraceptives			
Weight fluctuation in adult life exceeding 12kg			
Altered hunger tolerance in premenstruum			
Altered alcohol tolerance in premenstruum			

The effectiveness of the diagnostic checklist and of the SHBG estimation was tested on a group of 65 women consecutively attending the premenstrual clinic having been referred by their doctors with a diagnosis of premenstrual syndrome. Fig. 3.16 shows the scattergram of the diagnostic checklist scores and the SHBG result for the 42 women (65%) who had the diagnosis confirmed, compared with the 35% who were found to have some other diagnosis to account for their symptoms.

The sensitivity of the various items on the diagnostic checklist is shown in Table 3.5.

Consider the diagnostic pointers in an individual case. A 33-year-old housewife was charged with infanticide. She had drowned her baby in the bath and then taken an overdose. Questioning revealed that the incident had occurred the day before menstruation and she had eaten no food after breakfast at 0800. She is thought to have drowned the baby at about 1700 hours. Premenstrual syndrome had been present since puberty as

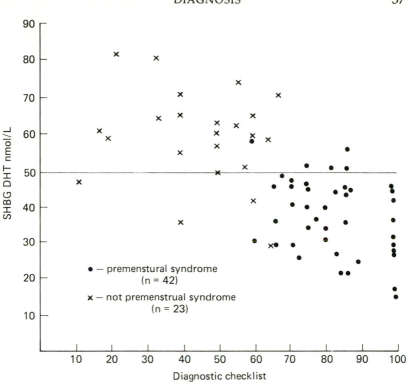

Fig. 3.16 Scattergram of SHBG and diagnostic checklist percentage.

Table 3.5

Effectiveness of diagnostic checklist

	PMS n=42	Not PMS n=23
	%	%
Time of onset	86	41*
Time of increased severity	100	0*
Painless menstruation	83	29*
Pregnancy (threatened abortion, pre-eclampsia/ postnatal depression)	76	50*
Oral contraceptives	81	50*
Weight fluctuations	65	25*
Altered hunger tolerance	96	66*
Altered alcohol tolerance	100	0*

*=Statistically significant at 5% level

shown on her medical records. Her first pregnancy had been complicated by pre-eclampsia. Her second pregnancy had been complicated by severe postpartum haemorrhage for which she had been admitted to an intensive care unit, and this had been followed by postnatal depression for which she had received treatment from a general practitioner and a psychiatrist. Her menstrual chart since the incident confirmed premenstrual syndrome. She was unable to tolerate the contraceptive pill, which caused depression and such a pronounced rise in blood pressure that she was admitted to hospital for investigation. She recognised that she became bad-tempered after long intervals without food. She abstained from alcohol. She was successful in her plea of premenstrual syndrome.

This is an example of the valuable information which can be obtained from careful history taking.

4

Differential diagnosis

Premenstrual syndrome is 'the recurrence of symptoms in the pre-menstruum with absence in the postmenstruum'.

The presence of premenstrual symptoms is not in itself definitive evidence of premenstrual syndrome for the innumerable symptoms to be found in premenstrual syndrome may also occur in men, children and postmenopausal women; hence, the possible differential diagnoses are limitless and cover the entire range of medicine. This chapter will deal with only the common differential diagnoses as seen in a busy premenstrual syndrome clinic, and these will be considered in the order in which they present – that is, at interview, general examination, vaginal examination and on completion of a menstrual chart.

Presenting symptom

If the presenting symptom also occurs in the postmenstruum, even to only a mild or moderate extent, then the patient is suffering from menstrual distress and the cause of her symptoms needs further investigation.

Depression may be due to an endogenous depression or *anxiety* due to neurosis; both conditions require further psychiatric evaluation.

Lethargy may require the exclusion of hypothyroidism by thyroid function tests, and hypokalaemia due to excessive diuretic intake, which can be confirmed by electrolyte estimation.

Bloatedness may be a manifestation of idiopathic oedema resulting from prolonged dieting, excessive diuretics and self-

Table 4.1

Schedule of differential diagnosis

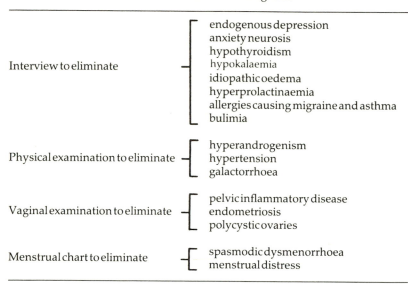

Interview to eliminate	endogenous depression anxiety neurosis hypothyroidism hypokalaemia idiopathic oedema hyperprolactinaemia allergies causing migraine and asthma bulimia
Physical examination to eliminate	hyperandrogenism hypertension galactorrhoea
Vaginal examination to eliminate	pelvic inflammatory disease endometriosis polycystic ovaries
Menstrual chart to eliminate	spasmodic dysmenorrhoea menstrual distress

imposed fluctuations of sodium and carbohydrate intake.

Breast tenderness and engorgement may result from hyper-prolactinaemia which can be confirmed by prolactin estimation.

Headaches and migraine may be caused by specific allergies or prolonged intervals between food.

Asthma may result from allergies, either inhaled or ingested. A common one seen in the premenstrual syndrome clinic is due to sensitivity to aspirin taken to alleviate some other premenstrual symptom such as backache.

Food cravings and compulsive eating may be a manifestation of excessive dieting or bulimia in one who has previously suffered from anorexia nervosa.

Physical examination

Hyperandrogenism may occur among disturbed and violent adolescents, who regularly shave their faces and wear jeans and long sleeves so that evidence of hirsutism is not suspected by the psychologists and social workers under whose care they come. Evidence of male hair distribution on the abdomen and buttocks, together with raised testosterone and androstendione levels confirm the diagnosis. Antitestosterone agents, such as cypro-terone acetate, give excellent results (Dalton, 1981).

Hypertension may account for headaches and anxiety.

Galactorrhoea may be evidence of *hyperprolactinaemia*, which requires further investigation to exclude a microadenoma of the pituitary.

Vaginal examination

Pain on moving the uterus may be due either to pelvic inflamma-tory disease, endometriosis or constipation. In *pelvic inflammatory disease* there may be evidence of a vaginal discharge, suprapubic pain, bilateral adenexal tenderness and sometimes a history of low-grade pyrexia. In *endometriosis* there may be a bulky uterus and a history of dyspareunia and infertility. *Constipation* will be apparent on vaginal examination with pain over the rectum and loaded faeces palpable in the pouch of Douglas.

Menstrual charts

When a patient returns with a menstrual chart completed for at least two months, three types of patterns are discernible.

1. *Premenstrual Syndrome* in which symptoms are grouped in the premenstruum with an absence of symptoms for a minimum of seven days in the postmenstruum (Fig. 3.5).
2. *Dysmenorrhoea* in which the symptoms are limited to menstruation and are absent in the premenstruum and postmenstruum (Fig. 4.1). In spasmodic dysmenorrhoea the symptoms are usually of pain, backache, and possibly vomiting or fainting (see Chapter 19).
3. *Menstrual distress* with symptoms occurring spasmodically throughout the cycle, but most marked in the paramen-struum (see Fig. 3.8).

Double diagnosis

It is, of course, possible to have premenstrual syndrome present at the same time as some other disease and so cause an exacerbation of the symptoms in the premenstruum. Depression is perhaps the most common example and if present throughout the cycle the diagnosis would be menstrual distress. However, it is important to recognise what proportion of symptoms are attributable to pre-menstrual syndrome and what proportion to the other disease, for only then can one estimate the degree of relief that may be

	Jan.	Feb.	March	April		May	June	July	Aug.
1									
2									
3									
4									
5									MX
6				MX					M
7		MX	MX	MX					
8		MX	MX	M					
9		MX	M	M					
10		M	M	M					
11		M	M						
12	MX	M							
13	MX								
14	MX								
15	M								
16	M								
17									
18									
19									
20									
21									
22						MX			
23						MX			
24						M			
25									
26									
27									
28							MX		
29							M		
30							M		
31									

M = menstruation

X = symptoms. (pain and backache)

Fig. 4.1 Two charts showing spasmodic dysmenorrhoea.

expected from progesterone in the treatment of premenstrual syndrome.

Figure 4.2 shows varying proportions of exacerbation of symptoms in the premenstruum. In pattern A the underlying disease accounts for 95% of the symptoms and there is only a slight increase of symptoms during the premenstruum. In contrast, pattern E shows that premenstrual syndrome forms an important component of the symptoms and the underlying

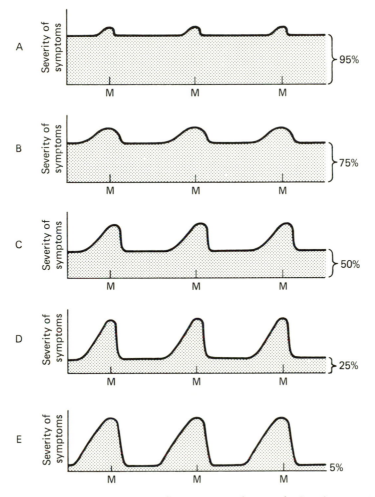

Fig. 4.2 Varying proportions of premenstrual exacerbation in menstrual distress.

disease is responsible for only 5% of the symptoms in the postmenstruum. Progesterone treatment of those with patterns C, D and E would seem to be justified, provided that both the medical attendant and the patient appreciate that such treatment will bring only partial benefit.

Occasionally the symptoms can be separated – for example, headaches occurring intermittently throughout the cycle and depression only in the premenstruum (Fig. 4.3). Here again the decision to treat the premenstrual component will depend on the proportion of the total symptoms, and there must be an appreciation that only premenstrual depression will be relieved by progesterone while the headaches will not be affected.

	Jan.	Feb.	March	April
1	X	X		
2	X	X		
3	X	X	H	
4	X	X		H
5	X	X		H
6	P	X		
7	P	X		
8	PH	X		
9	P	X	X	
10		X	X	H
11		PX	X	
12		P	X	
13		PH	X	
14	H	P	X	H
15		P	X	
16			X	
17			PX	
18		H	PX	
19			PH	X
20			P	HX
21			P	X
22			P	X
23				X
24				X
25	H			X
26				XP
27		H		XP
28		H		P
29				P
30				P
31				

X = depression
H = headache

Fig. 4.3   Premenstrual depression with intermittent headaches.

5

Symptomatology

Premenstrual syndrome is 'the recurrence of symptoms in the pre-menstruum with absence in the postmenstruum'.

Symptoms that can occur in the syndrome are of extraordinary diversity and include many of the commonest symptoms of each medical speciality (Table 5.1). It seems that no tissues in the body are exempt from the cyclical changes of the menstrual cycle, and all can be affected by cyclical premenstrual symptoms or exacerbations of chronic disorders.

The symptoms present at the first visit of 610 patients seen in 1982 are shown in Table 5.2, while Table 5.3 compares their symptoms with those of the 86 patients with premenstrual syndrome reported by Greene and Dalton in 1953. In the recent study the symptoms were predominantly psychological ones with few eye, ear, nose, throat or skin lesions. This is not necessarily the true incidence of symptoms, but merely reflects the psychological orientation of doctors and the public. Those working in specialised clinics, who have been alerted to the possibility of premenstrual syndrome, soon recognise examples of premenstrual syndrome and note their response to progesterone therapy. (See Appendix Tables 27.4 & 27.5.)

The psychological symptoms of premenstrual tension, with its depression, irritability and lethargy, are undoubtedly the commonest and it is possible that tension is always present, even if overshadowed by more serious presenting symptoms, such as asthma, epilepsy or migraine. A housewife presented with a minor stye on her upper lid and added 'I can't put up with these

45

Table 5.1

Common symptoms of premenstrual syndrome

Psychological	Tension Depression Irritability Lethargy
Neurological	Migraine Epilepsy Syncope
Dermatological	Acne Herpes Urticaria
Respiratory	Asthma Rhinitis
Orthopaedic	Joint pains Backache
Opthalmalogical	Glaucoma Conjunctivitis Styes
Otolaryngorhinological	Sinusitis Sore throats

much longer, they make me feel so ill I feel exhausted and have headaches for two days before, and I am ready to take my life.' The visible symptom was covering up the invisible distress of premenstrual syndrome.

Polysymptomatology

One characteristic is the tendency for the patient to be poly-symptomatic with an increasing accumulation of symptoms reaching a crescendo on the final day of the premenstruum. Frequent combinations are tension, headache and mastitis, or depression, backache and nausea. The symptoms do not necessarily all start at the same time. A woman may wake up one morning feeling the world is against her, tired yet making an effort to get up and carry on with the normal routine. A couple of days later she may be conscious of painfully engorged breasts, and

Table 5.2

Symptoms at first visit

	n=610	
	n	%
Depression	435	71
Irritability	343	56
Tiredness	212	35
Headaches	202	33
Bloatedness	188	31
Breast tenderness	129	21
Tension	115	19
Violence	80	13
Suicidal	36	6
Anxiety/panics	33	5
Food cravings	30	5
Criminal acts	22	4
Epilepsy	19	3
Psychotic episodes	17	3
Skin lesions	17	3
Vertigo	16	3
Alcoholic urges	13	2
Asthma	9	1.5
Urinary symptoms	6	1
Ear, nose and throat lesions	4	0.7
Eye lesions	4	0.7

Table 5.3

Comparison of premenstrual syndrome in 1953 and 1982

	Greene and Dalton %	*1982* %
Headache	69	33
Irritability	30	56
Depression	6	71
Lethargy	6	35
Vertigo	13	3
Skin and mucosal	13	3
Oedema/bloatedness	6	31
Rhinitis	7	1
Asthma	5	1
Epilepsy	5	3
Mastalgia	2	21

realise that she is irritable with the children. Gradually she develops a headache, which increases in severity over the next 12 or 24 hours until she is prostrated with photophobia, vomiting and with a throbbing hemicranial headache. With the onset of menstruation her migraine eases and so do her other symptoms.

The timing of symptoms

The common time patterns of symptoms are shown in Fig. 2.1. Frequently symptoms have been present for a few days before they become incapacitating. Analysis of absenteeism due to sickness among women employees in a light engineering factory and in a multiple store showed that 45% occurred during the eight days of the paramenstruum, compared with an expected incidence of 29% expected on an even distribution (Dalton, 1964).

In many women there is often a day or two of slight menstrual bleeding before the onset of the full menstrual flow, and it is not uncommon among these women to find symptoms persisting through the first few days of the cycle.

Onset of symptoms

Symptoms often start abruptly on waking in the morning. The woman may state that she 'feels different' or that she 'knows the kind of day it'll be'. There is then an increase in the number of different symptoms, such as headache, backache, oedema, until they reach a crescendo on about day 28 or day 1. On the other hand, onset may be preceded by a day of restless activity or hypermania which is later blamed for the onset of her attack. The husband has often heard her say that she does too much and brings on her own attacks. One patient described how, 'I do mountains of housework, then suddenly it all changes', and another, 'I'm a bundle of restless energy until it starts'.

The ending of symptoms

Symptoms ease after the onset of the full menstrual flow, but the ending of symptoms varies in each individual according to the time, during menstruation, when they experience the full menstrual flow. Furthermore, the type of ending of symptoms may change in any individual during her menstruating life.

There are those who have an abrupt ending of symptoms, as described in such phrases as 'a cloud lifts', 'like a switch it's gone' and 'suddenly my head clears and I know I will be all right'. These are women who experience the full menstrual flow on the first day, and then the flow may either continue to be heavy until the end, as in pattern A1, Fig. 5.1, or it may lessen after a day or two as in pattern A2. On the other hand, there are those women who have a slight menstrual loss for one or more days before the full menstrual flow, and they will not have relief until the second day of menstruation or later (patterns B1 and B2, Fig. 5.1). Indeed, their symptoms may be worse during the days of light menstrual loss. This pattern of menstruation often occurs after the insertion of an intrauterine device.

In some cases the pathological process started in the pre-menstruum may take a few days to resolve – for example, acne, herpes.

Transition of symptoms

Over the years there may be a gradual transition of the main symptoms, particularly when the normal course of premenstrual syndrome has been interrupted with a pregnancy.

Premenstrual rhinitis may gradually be replaced by pre-menstrual asthma. Premenstrual backache may later present as mastitis, with backache as a secondary symptom, and gradually abdominal bloatedness may be more important although engorged breasts and backache are still present.

Effect of stress

As with all hormonal diseases, at times of stress the symptoms of premenstrual syndrome are increased in severity and number. The mild and easily controlled tension or headache, otherwise relieved by a simple analgesic, may suddenly be exacerbated and additional symptoms become manifest at times of redundancy, bereavement or financial embarrassment or whenever life becomes intolerable. A fortunate win at the pools was known to cure one housewife of premenstrual asthma, which later returned when she was covering up for her son's delinquency.

The influence of stress may come to light if, when taking a full medical history, a special note is made of the times of previous illnesses, particularly previous investigations of the same symptoms and keeping these events in mind when taking a social history. This was demonstrated in a mother of four children who came with a good menstrual record showing premenstrual backache and headaches, which she stated had been present since

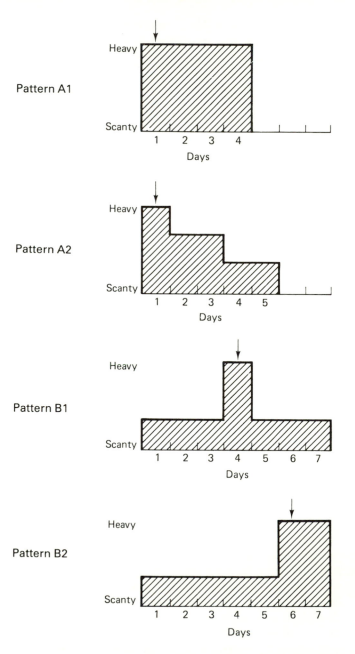

Fig. 5.1 Times of heaviest menstrual flow.

the birth of her first child. She had previously attended the neurological clinic for investigation of her headaches at the time she moved into a new house. Four years later she attended the orthopaedic clinic for investigations and physiotherapy shortly after both parents had been killed in a road accident. Her sinuses were examined by x-ray at the same time as her husband was in hospital having a gastrectomy. Thus stress caused her chronic premenstrual symptoms to become unbearable and she demanded treatment at these times.

It must be remembered that stress can also alter the length of cycle or duration of blood loss as well as increasing the severity of premenstrual symptoms. This was illustrated in an analysis of the days of menstruation of 91 boarding school girls, aged 16 years, who were taking their 'O' level examinations at the same time. Whereas an average of 16 girls were menstruating on any one day during the month of May, on one day during the stress of examination week in June as many as 36 girls were menstruating (Fig. 5.2) (Dalton, 1968).

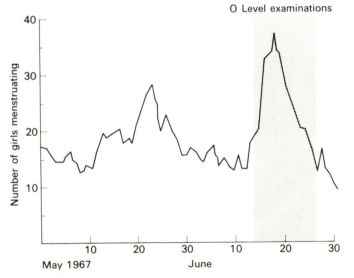

Fig. 5.2   Time of menstruation of 91 examination candidates. (From Dalton K. (1968). *Lancet*; **ii**:1386.)

Site of symptom

The site of the predominant symptom may be localised in relation to the patient's current occupation. In 1954 during a survey into the incidence of premenstrual syndrome in the general population, part of the investigation was carried out in a light engineering factory employing some 3000 women. Batches of about 20 women were interviewed each day, and it was noted that on some days complaints of backache predominated while on other days headaches were a common symptom. Then it was learned that the women were released from one department at a time. Those complaining predominantly of premenstrual backache were employed in the packing department where the work entailed standing and lifting, while those with premenstrual headaches sat all day at a bench under strong light assembling minute parts, a task requiring a high level of concentration and visual acuity (Dalton, 1954).

Exacerbation of chronic diseases in the premenstruum

Many chronic diseases have a premenstrual exacerbation and it is characteristically those diseases which usually improve during pregnancy: examples include rheumatoid arthritis, endogenous depression, ulcerative colitis, asthma and peptic ulcer. Deterioration in mitral stenosis as evidenced by increasing dyspnoea, haemoptysis, oedema and signs of right ventricular failure have been noted to increase during the premenstruum with distinct improvement during the postmenstruum. It is because of the possibility of chronic disease being present that it must be emphasised again that in premenstrual syndrome there is always a phase free from all symptoms during the postmenstruum.

Similarity of premenstrual symptoms to symptoms in pre-eclampsia

Among women who develop pre-eclampsia 87% subsequently suffer from the premenstrual syndrome regardless of whether the premenstrual syndrome had its onset before or after the affected pregnancy. It is usual for each individual to experience the same symptoms both during the premenstruum and during the affected pregnancy. Thus one woman may be afflicted by occipital headaches and backache, and another by vertigo and paraesthesia of her hands and feet. This is shown in Fig. 5.3 giving the pattern of premenstrual and pregnancy symptoms experienced by 191 sufferers from pre-eclampsia, compared with 169 controls and 87 women who suffered from the premenstrual syndrome but had experienced normal pregnancies (Dalton, 1954).

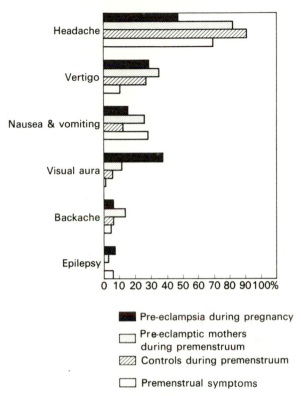

Fig. 5.3 Symptoms present during pre-eclampsia and the premenstruum.

Mechanisms of symptoms

The wide diversity of symptoms manifested in premenstrual syndrome can be grouped into six functions of progesterone or of the adrenohypothalamic-pituitary-ovarian pathway (Table 5.4).

1. Relative hypoglycaemia.
2. Water retention.
3. Potassium depletion and sodium retention.
4. Allergic reactions.
5. Lowered resistance to infections.
6. Inflammatory reactions.

Relative hypoglycaemia

As long ago as 1925 Okey and Robb reported – and it has been confirmed by other workers – that, during menstruation, fasting

Table 5.4

Symptomology of premenstrual syndrome

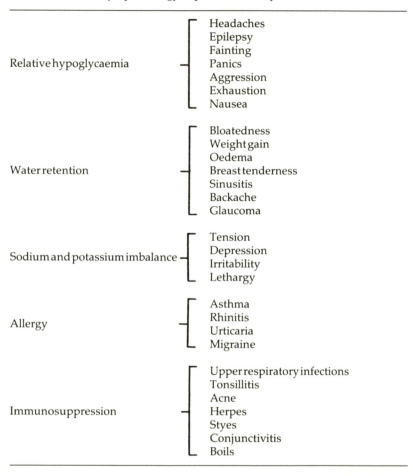

Relative hypoglycaemia	Headaches Epilepsy Fainting Panics Aggression Exhaustion Nausea
Water retention	Bloatedness Weight gain Oedema Breast tenderness Sinusitis Backache Glaucoma
Sodium and potassium imbalance	Tension Depression Irritability Lethargy
Allergy	Asthma Rhinitis Urticaria Migraine
Immunosuppression	Upper respiratory infections Tonsillitis Acne Herpes Styes Conjunctivitis Boils

blood sugar levels were higher and glucose tolerance levels were flattened. It seems that this altered carbohydrate tolerance is responsible not only for the food cravings and ravenous appetite in the premenstruum, but also for many other symptoms, including the acute attacks which characterise this syndrome, such as sudden loss of control resulting in panic attacks, fainting, epilepsy, and migraine (Billig & Spalding). To appreciate fully how this operates one needs to understand the two regulating mechanisms which maintain blood glucose level within normal limits, and which break down in diabetes (Fig. 5.4). If too much carbohydrate is ingested the blood glucose level rises until it reaches the upper regulating mechanisms and the renal threshold when the excess glucose is excreted in the urine. Similarly if there

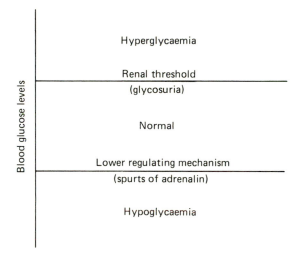

Fig. 5.4 Control mechanism for blood glucose.

is no carbohydrate intake the level of glucose falls until it reaches the lower regulating mechanism. This operates by giving a spurt of adrenaline which causes the release of glucose from the cells to raise the blood glucose level. If no further carbohydrate is ingested the blood glucose will again fall and there will be further spurts of adrenaline until the next carbohydrate-containing meal. In the premenstruum, and particularly among sufferers of pre-menstrual syndrome, the lower regulating mechanism is raised, so the individual is not able to go as long before the regulator comes into action and a spurt of adrenaline occurs. Many of the sudden explosive attacks of aggression, panic, migraine and epilepsy tend to occur when there has been a long interval without food (Fig. 5.5).

It should be appreciated that these are not attacks of hypoglycaemia as the blood sugar level never drops to hypo-glycaemic levels, and a normal three-hour oral glucose tolerance test will be normal.

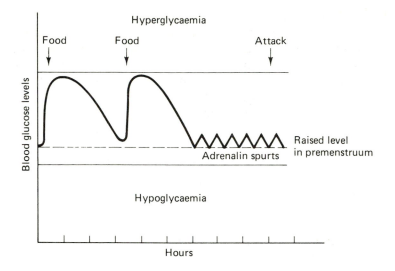

Fig. 5.5   Effect of long interval without food in the premenstruum in sufferers of premenstrual syndrome.

The use of attack forms (see Fig 3.12) is particularly valuable in recognising those attacks which appear to be related to long intervals between food. By obtaining a detailed history of food intake before an attack it is possible to differentiate those cases where an interval of five or more hours without food has occurred.

There is often a natural temptation to diet and limit food intake at a time of premenstrual weight gain and abdominal bloatedness. An unmarried mother of a 6-year-old girl was referred by the social agencies because she had battered her child; the last two occasions were noted as being during the premenstruum. During the interview she stated that she always felt more irritable in the late afternoon when her child returned from school. Further questioning revealed that apart from her bran at breakfast she would not eat any food until teatime. During her premenstruum she could not tolerate long intervals without food.

Another group at risk are young teenagers who, after an early supper, have an energetic evening dancing, skating or swimming before going to bed without further food; they then rush off to work next morning with no time for breakfast. They are liable to transient attacks of relative hypoglycaemia.

Water retention

Water retention is not necessarily present in premenstrual syndrome. Several studies of patients with premenstrual syndrome and normal controls have shown that there are no significant weight changes related to the premenstruum between the two groups. The symptoms may be due to a redistribution of fluid, with an increased flow from the intravascular to the extracellular compartments, certain tissues being more sensitive than others to slight alterations. (Lamb *et al.*, Dalton 1954 & 1967, Klein & Carey, Chesley, Fortin *et al.*, Appleby, Bruce & Russell.)

The water retention may be associated with the relative hypoglycaemia, but it is generally considered that retention is the effect of progesterone deficiency on the renin-angiotensin-aldosterone axis. Progesterone stimulates an increase in plasma renin activity and increases aldosterone secretion and excretion.

High sodium or monosodium gluconate intake also causes water retention and is likely to occur in those whose diet is high in convenience foods and savoury snacks.

Water retention is responsible for such symptoms as oedema of the ankles, bloated abdomen, puffy face, engorged breasts, nasal obstruction, sinusitis, headache and eye pain. It is suggested by the oliguria and weight gain which precede an attack and the spontaneous diuresis and weight loss which mark the end of an attack. The water retention may be local or general, and only if it is general will it be recognised by weight gain. On the other hand, only a minute increase in the amount of aqueous humour is required to cause a rise in intraocular pressure, an amount that is not necessarily revealed by the omnibus method of weighing the whole patient.

Localisation of water retention may be manifested in three ways.

1. Acute symptoms from localised oedema, as with migraine or epilepsy, sinus headache, vertigo due to oedema in the labyrinth, and pruritis from subcutaneous oedema.
2. Vague symptoms resulting from widespread distribution as in abdominal bloating and generalised heaviness.
3. A gain in weight without any symptoms can occur, especially in the obese when the fluid is distributed in the fat and subcutaneous tissue.

In many surveys a weight gain during the premenstruum has

been observed in those with or without symptoms, this has been falsely interpreted as meaning that water retention is not an important factor in premenstrual syndrome. In many women water retention is important and they benefit from diuretics, but the danger of diuretic addiction should not be overlooked. There are other factors responsible for the premenstrual symptoms in those who do not show a weight gain and such patients do not benefit from diuretics.

The actual site of the oedematous cells may vary from time to time, factors which determine their location may include the following:

1. Anatomy. A sinus headache is more likely to occur if, in addition to engorged mucus membrane, there is a deflected septum; and a closed angle at the anterior chamber of the eye can interfere with the normal outflow of ocular fluid.
2. Heredity, as with a family history of epilepsy. An anatomical abnormality may also be inherited.
3. Injury. Fluid is readily attracted to a site that has recently been oedematous as a result of injury, such as a fractured wrist or ankle, and for many months there may be a tendency for premenstrual oedema to recur at the site of the old injury.
4. Infection. Following pneumonia there may be recurrent premenstrual dyspnoea for the next few months, as cells which have recently been inflamed easily become oedematous.

Potassium depletion and sodium retention

It is the imbalance of potassium and sodium which is responsible for the tension symptoms of lethargy, muscle weakness, irritability and depression. Diuretics which help symptoms due to water retention, do not remove the tension symptoms and, indeed, may increase symptoms by causing hypokalaemia and increased lethargy and irritability. At the peak of premenstrual tension one may find a low potassium concentration, and indeed such patients will benefit from potassium supplement to raise their potassium from the lower level of normal range to an optimum of 4.0 to 4.3 mmol/1.

Allergy, lowered resistance to infection and inflammatory reactions

Progesterone is an immunosuppressive agent (Rothchild). Its prime function occurs during pregnancy, when the progesterone concentration is greatly raised and when its function is to protect the mother from the fetus growing within her uterus. It is possible that the premenstrual allergic manifestations of asthma, rhinitis, urticaria and migraine occur when progesterone is required by the endometrium and there is insufficient for systemic immuno-suppression. The same applies to evidence of lowered resistance to infection and the increased inflammatory reactions occurring during the premenstruum in some women. This would account for the recurrent premenstrual tonsillitis, sinusitis, acne, styes, boils, herpes and conjunctivitis.

6

Psychological symptoms

Premenstrual syndrome is 'the recurrence of symptoms in the premenstruum with absence in the postmenstruum'.

In 1959 a survey of four London hospitals showed that of 276 emergency psychiatric admissions 46% had occurred during the paramenstruum (Fig. 6.1) (Dalton).

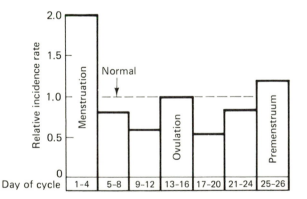

Fig. 6.1   Time of acute psychiatric admission in 276 patients. (From Dalton K. (1959). *Br. Med. J.*; **1**:148–149.)

Indeed 53% of attempted suicides, 47% of admissions for depression and 47% of schizophrenic patients were admitted during these eight days of the menstrual cycle (Figs. 6.2; 6.3; 6.4).

Similar surveys throughout the world have tended to produce

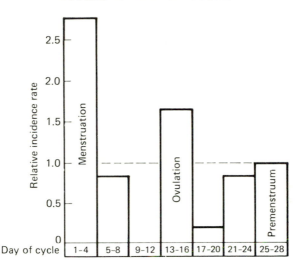

Fig. 6.2   Time of menstrual cycle of 36 attempted suicides. (From Dalton K. (1959) *Br. Med. J.*; **1**:148–149.)

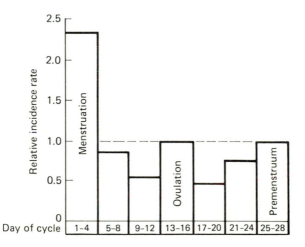

Fig. 6.3   Time of admission of 185 patients with depression. (From Dalton K. (1959). *Br. Med. J.*; **1**:148–149.)

much the same results. Abramowitz and his colleagues (1982) have recently confirmed these findings and have also shown that among depressed women (but not among a comparison group of schizophrenic women) there is a pronounced rise in admission

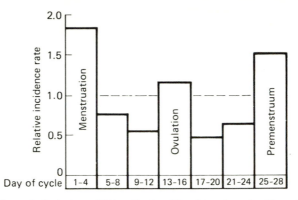

Fig. 6.4 Time of admission of 114 patients with schizophrenia. (From Dalton K. (1959). *Br. Med. J.*; 1:148–149.)

frequency on the last day of the premenstruum and the first day of menstruation. Of the depressed women, 41% admitted during the paramenstruum were admitted on these two particular days compared with an expected 25% of admissions if there had been an even distribution of admissions throughout the eight paramenstrual days.

The incidence of psychological symptoms is shown in Tables 5.2, 27.4 & 27.5. Many of the women had more than one presenting symptom.

Premenstrual tension

The commonest symptom of premenstrual syndrome is tension, which is recognised as having three components: *depression, irritability* and *lethargy* (Tables 27.7 & 27.25). Indeed it is likely that few cases of premenstrual syndrome are seen in which tension is not also present, although it is easy enough to blame the presenting symptom – for example, asthma or epilepsy – for causing the tension. In 1953 Billig aptly described the tension as 'the world looks like a sour apple', 'crabbiness' and 'a fall in energy'. Tension may be so acute and disabling that in France, for example, it is recognised for legal purposes as temporary insanity. On the other hand, in its mildest form, it may be no more than the natural change of emotions.

Mood swings

The most characteristic symptom is the sudden mood swing.

A woman may be conversing genially when suddenly, for no obvious reason, she becomes uncontrollably argumentative and aggressive and is indeed a 'changed personality'. A 35-year-old teacher married to a headmaster stated: 'For seven days during the premenstruum I became tense, shouting, irritable, weepy, tired, bloated with a swelling of legs and ankles and with headaches over the eyes. I have had two children and at those times when in an uncontrollable temper I have hit them really hard.' She was successfully treated with progesterone for 12 months and has been free from symptoms ever since. She later wrote: 'It has been a valuable experience – I would never have believed that an intelligent woman like me, with high morals and good education could ever lose control of herself to such an extent that she would batter her children, for I love my children dearly. How utterly illogical it is that I personally should cause them permanent damage.'

The suddenness of this change in personality is something men rarely experience. At a recent medical meeting, however, a doctor with diabetes, stabilised on insulin, discussed his disease. To him the most distressing part was his inability to control his own emotions when the aggressive and quarrelsome outbursts occurred unexpectedly when he suddenly became hypoglycaemic. There are many women with premenstrual syndrome who would sympathise with him in his inability to be master of his own emotions. So often a woman finds a sudden rage within her which changes her from a placid personality into an irritable, aggressive, irrational, nagging female.

Depression

Depression is manifested by weeping and a pessimistic outlook, easily relieved by congenial company. Although it may be severe, the duration is seldom more than a few days, 14 at most. The survey of 610 women with premenstrual syndrome (Table 5.2) and Tables 27.2 & 27.3 in the Appendix showed that at the first visit depression was the commonest symptom, occurring in 71–73% of them, being highest in nulliparous women.

While the premenstrual depression lasts it has all the characteristics of endogenous depression with the loss of interest and enthusiasm, forgetfulness, indecision, tearfulness, guilt, inability to concentrate, with feelings of insecurity and inadequacy, lack of insight and exhaustion. It differs, however, in that the combination of irritability, irrationality and impatience is a prominent feature, there is weight gain instead of weight loss, food cravings instead of anorexia, and hypersomnia may occur instead of insomnia with early morning waking. The most marked difference is the short duration which can be measured in days instead of weeks or months, and there is a definite beginning and ending to each episode.

The depression may vary from feeling bored and jaded with a 'can't be bothered' attitude, to uncontrollable tears and life-threatening situations. The woman feels inferior, nobody loves her and she is upset by the least thing, making mountains out of molehills.

One woman wrote, 'I want to back into a corner and stay there undisturbed like a mouse'.

Another woman wrote: 'My problem is, about ten days before my period comes, I get uncontrollable fits of depression which makes me hit rock bottom. If I am with a crowd of friends I feel like I am going to suffocate. It is a feeling which comes over me and I want to run out. The same thing seems to happen with me if I am with one person. All I want to do is cry and my mind thinks of all morbid things possible. Also a very strong feeling of loneliness comes over me which makes me feel I am choking with fear. I am usually a normal woman of 28 years who has plenty of friends who I get on with very well and in general people seem to like me. But as I said before, about a week and a half before the period comes my whole personality seems to change and I feel that I can't go on much longer like this, it drains all energy from me.'

Those close to the sufferer are likely to recognise her moods; the husband will know this is not an opportune moment to discuss the family budget, and the office staff will avoid making plans, suggesting alterations or asking favours.

Another woman described the change as being like 'from Dr Jekyll to Mr Hyde, I become subject to depression, feel emotionally unstable, hysterical and miserable. Sometimes I get so keyed up that I can't sleep for 2 or 3 days before a period starts. I feel pressure across the base of my skull as if my brain was swollen.'

Tears are always near the surface during the premenstruum in many women, as noted by McCance et al. Their findings are shown in Fig. 6.5.

One woman gave up driving on certain days because she

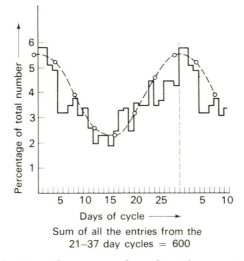

Fig. 6.5 Variation in tendency to cry throughout the menstrual cycle. (From McCance R.A., Luff M.C., Widdowson E.E. (1938). *J. Hyg.*; **37**:571–611.)

tended to burst into tears each time the traffic lights were against her. Another recalled 'sitting in the theatre with tears rolling down my cheeks – squeezing my hands and saying to myself "No – I musn't, this is a comedy – everyone else is laughing".'

The depression is especially marked in teenagers and meno-pausal women, and in both these groups, if charts are kept they may well show monthly mood swings at times of missed menstruation as well as at menstruation. One may suspect an underlying depression if the sufferer blames some minor ailment – such as a boil – for the lethargy and malaise, creating the impression that if only this one small spot would disappear all the mental tension would go.

Suicides

About half of all attempted and successful suicides in women occur during the paramenstruum. This has been confirmed by surveys as far apart as London, Los Angeles and Delhi (Gregory, Dalton, MacKinnon & MacKinnon, Ribero, Wetzel & McClure, Devi & Rao). Although women make more attempts at suicide than men, the men succeed more frequently, although this success rate in men disappears after the age of 50 years. Dr John

Pollitt, speaking at the Royal Society of Medicine, London, in 1976 suggested that:

> 'Perhaps one reason for the female's lack of success is that the majority of attempts are made during the premenstrual phase or menstruation. Killing oneself is not easy; success requires careful planning. Women in the premenstrual phase show a marked tendency to be careless, thoughtless, unpunctual, forgetful and absentminded. This inefficiency at a time when they are more likely to try and end their lives may result in a disproportionate failure.'

While it is possible that some suicides may be attributed solely to premenstrual syndrome, it seems that in most cases there is an underlying endogenous depression in which the additional burden of premenstrual depression acts as a trigger to increase the severity until breaking point is reached. Suicidal attempts due solely to premenstrual syndrome are characteristically preceded by a quarrel and are not premeditated; with the onset of menstruation these patients rapidly recover from their depression. Witnesses will confirm that the woman was her usual happy, vivacious self until an hour or two before the attempt. The quarrel is usually about something very unimportant – a typical storm in a teacup.

A 30-year-old housewife, whose premenstrual syndrome was recognised when she was a teenager and became worse after marriage when she started on the pill, found that during the seven premenstrual days she was irritable and tense, more aggressive and violent (often self-directed as well as directed towards husband and elder child). During the premenstruum she 'over-reacted' to stress and became more emotional. On the first day of menstruation all symptoms eased and she became calm, friendly and rational. She was unable to tolerate the contraceptive pill, which caused depression. During her pregnancies she became free from mood swings and 'happy' but had puerperal depression. She had made five suicidal gestures, each one on the last premenstrual day with an overdose of aspirin; an overdose of Valium; slashing her wrist; self-stabbing; and jumping under a train. On 16 March she lost her temper and hit her elder daughter aged five years who would not stop crying. She was then shocked by her action and asked for her children to be taken into care.

Menstruation started on 18 March. On progesterone therapy she became symptom free.

While suicide gestures are recognised as cries for help and a longing for love, there are other ways in which some women try to achieve this. In some, the attention-seeking episode results in them slashing their wrists, shaving their heads, arson, or making unnecessary emergency telephone calls to the fire station or police. These, too, may be at monthly intervals as shown in the above case history and illustrated in the two case histories in Chapter 3. Although the urge for the premenstrual attention-seeking gesture may be shortlived the results may be lifelong, as with the scars on the wrists for which plastic surgery is later requested, permanent kidney or liver damage resulting from massive overdoses, a permanent limp from jumping from a fifth floor window or a paralysed arm from a leap on to the railway line.

Irritability

Irritability can cover the whole range from the cross word or sarcastic remark to quarrels with abusive slanging and swearing, to slamming doors and throwing things, to violence which knows no bounds and ends in actual bodily harm or even murder. A feature of premenstrual tension is the loss of control in those who normally would not raise their voices or assert themselves.

Irritability was mentioned at the first visit by 61% of the women with premenstrual syndrome reported in Table 5.2 (Dalton, 1982).

The irritability is irrational and usually accompanied by little insight. Patients will describe themselves as 'agitated – jittery – intolerant – impatient – spiteful – fault finding – vindictive – irrational – snappy – screaming – shouting – nagging – useless – bitchy – the least thing upsets me – the children won't behave – frightening to the children – I try not to shout at the children – quarrelsome – quick-tempered – I can't suffer fools gladly'. Often the incident which provokes the anger has been present for some time, but suddenly the woman explodes with anger over some triviality like a coat lying on the floor, or a missing button on her husband's jacket (Fig. 6.6).

The sudden fiery outburst of irritability may be similar to the psychomotor attacks of epilepsy, and could be lightly dismissed as hysteria. Irritable outbursts are likely to occur when the woman has not eaten for some considerable time and may result from relative hypoglycaemia.

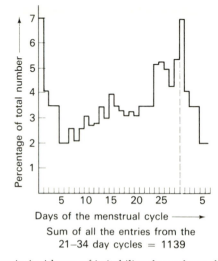

Fig. 6.6   Variation in incidence of irritability throughout the menstrual cycle. (From McCance R.A., Luff M.C., Widdowson E.E. (1938). *J. Hyg.*; **37:**571–611.)

During an outburst of irritability the woman may become violent and be prone to hit out at anyone within reach, often the nearest and dearest. She is generally completely unaware of the seriousness of her actions and is unable to prevent them. It is in these circumstances that the husband and/or children can and do get battered. The following case history of a 31-year-old secretary is all too common.

The premenstrual syndrome started after second childbirth. During the seven premenstrual days the woman became increasingly depressed and tense, and by the third premenstrual day became very irritable so that she might hit out at her daughters aged four and one year if they failed to obey her command instantly. She would wake up later to find herself crying and would then realise what harm she had done. She would become so exhausted that she would spend whole days in bed. The irritability eased with the onset of menstruation, and the depression and exhaustion slowly disappeared during the six days of menstruation. She was calm and energetic from day 6 to 16 of each cycle. She had two court appearances for assault on her children. She flew from Milan monthly for consultations and became free from premenstrual symptoms on progesterone.

Considering the number of mothers referred for treatment of the premenstrual syndrome, who are known to have battered their own children, the overall incidence of premenstrual battering must be very high but there have been no surveys into this aspect of non-accidental injuries.

Often the husband describes how he knows he will be unable to do anything right and that his wife will lose her usual understanding and become a 'nagger' or 'bitch' for a few days. It is also at this time that the employee will suddenly leave her job after a disagreement. The Industrial Tribunal has ruled that it is unfair to dismiss a female employee who has a premenstrual tantrum. Most marriage guidance counsellors are aware of the ill consequence that can arise from premenstrual irritability and will draw the attention of both members of the marriage partnership to the relationship of quarrelling to the menstrual cycle. The wise counsellor, when telephoned urgently at the time of a marital quarrel, will arrange a meeting for seven days later when the woman is likely to be in her calm postmenstrual phase.

The irritability may ease quite suddenly. It may be replaced by a sense of guilt at the trouble the tantrums have caused. As one woman said, 'I wish others would realise it wasn't the true me who caused all this'.

In the treatment of premenstrual tension, if a sub-optimal dose of progesterone is given in the first course it is most likely to bring the greatest relief to the irritability rather than to the depression or lethargy. As the dose is increased the depression is usually relieved before the lethargy.

Lethargy

Lethargy is both mental and physical, varying from a mild physiological tiredness to an overpowering desire to sleep. The woman may even feel 'too lazy to talk'. It is a lethargy that is difficult to overcome, resulting in slower piecetime work in the factory, impaired efficiency in the office and difficulty in composing letters, while teachers find themselves slower at marking homework and less able to maintain discipline. One teacher admitted 'every month there are one or two days when I am simply not worth the salary my employers pay me'. More than one secretary has been referred by her employer who noticed those few days each month when typing errors got out of control and the wastepaper basket was filled to overflowing. There is a desire to perform the minimum of work and an inability to cope with even routine jobs. Creative workers may notice a lack of inspiration and should postpone more important assignments until the lethargy has passed. Manual dexterity is lost and the resultant clumsiness may lead to unnecessary breakages. Paramenstrual lethargy must be widespread in the population or it would not appear so clearly in studies of mental ability and work performance (Chapter 21).

In its most severe form lethargy is seen in the woman who seeks refuge on the park bench on her way to work and sleeps there, or the housewife who sneaks up to bed once the family has gone to work or school. A 16-year-old girl at a boarding school was referred after the matron had found her sleeping at her desk while other girls were out playing (Dalton, 1964).

Alcohol excess

Belfer & Carroll noted that 67% of menstruating female alcoholics related their drinking bouts to their menstrual cycle and 100% indicated that drinking had begun or increased in the premenstruum. Women are more prone to alcoholic bouts, known to the agencies as 'once-a-monthers', compared with men, who tend to be chronic alcoholics indulging excessively every day. A woman who appeared in the television programme 'Pull Yourself Together Woman' was referred by the alcoholic agency after she had required three hospital admissions at monthly intervals for a suicide attempt and two self-inflicted injuries. She responded to progesterone therapy and was shown on television attending ballet classes after she had started her new life.

Alcohol appears to be more intoxicating during the paramenstruum when water retention is present. This, together with a premenstrual lack of self-control and depression, causes many women to have a monthly drinking bout, often in secret. During an investigation in prison, several women were noted to have a record of imprisonment at monthly intervals for being drunk and disorderly. One prisoner described how she always seemed to start menstruation in the police cell shortly after her arrest. The lack of self-control at this time of the menstrual cycle is seen in the following statements: 'I can understand all the dangers, and can control myself for about three weeks, and then it gets the better of me and I don't want to help myself any more.' 'I only take alcohol when I am depressed but I hate myself for doing it.'

Psychosis

Short-lived premenstrual psychotic episodes can occur, particularly after recovery from puerperal psychosis. It may take the form of delusions, hallucinations, distortion phenomena or feelings of unreality, which last for only a few days with complete recovery except for an amnesia or clouding of the affected days. One woman described it as 'living in a balloon, unable to reach anyone'. There may also be a premenstrual increase in an established psychotic illness leading to emergency hospital admission, as mentioned at the beginning of the chapter (see also Appendix and Table 27.20).

Nymphomania

Nymphomania in the premenstruum was noted by Israel in 1938, and Hart reported in 1960 that among normal women many experienced increased libido before menstruation. This phenomenon is especially troublesome in adolescent girls, who run away from home to follow the boys and are later taken into care when they are beyond their parents' control. Their nymphomania continues and each premenstruum they still attempt to escape: when found they are likely to be with male company in the park or cafés. Their response to progesterone treatment is most effective.

This can also be a problem in marriage, the woman having the highest sex urge at the times when she is most disagreeable and most irritable with her husband. It is a point that marriage guidance counsellors should bear in mind.

Phobias

The first acute phobic attack often occurs during a relative hypoglycaemic episode in the premenstruum, but how the phobias continue after that depends more on the handling of the initial attack than on the time relationship to the menstrual cycle. When the patient is receiving behaviour therapy consideration should be given to the phase of the cycle.

Disturbances of sleep

Sleep disturbances are common, either hypersomnia where the woman has the greatest difficulty in getting up in the morning even after 12 hours' sleep, or as insomnia with sleep being disturbed by dreams and nightmares. The sleep disturbance frequently precedes premenstrual tension by two or three days. If a hypnotic is given it is likely to increase the premenstrual lethargy.

7

Somatic symptoms and signs

Premenstrual syndrome is 'the recurrence of symptoms in the pre-
menstruum with absence of symptoms in the postmenstruum'.

Every system and probably every tissue of the body is affected
by changes in menstrual hormone concentrations. The symptoms
and signs of premenstrual syndrome are not limited to menstruating women but may occur in postmenopausal women, men and
children. Some conditions, which are included in the definition of
premenstrual syndrome and have symptoms limited to the
premenstruum, may have an underlying pathological process
continuing throughout the menstrual cycle. Examples of this
might include haemorrhoids or varicose veins, in which symptoms in the early stages may be limited to the premenstruum, but
as the disease progresses the stage is reached at which symptoms
occur throughout the cycle although there may be an exacerbation
of symptoms premenstrually. Such conditions represent menstrual distress in an underlying disease. The somatic symptoms
discussed in this chapter may in different individuals represent
premenstrual syndrome or menstrual distress, or even a double
diagnosis of premenstrual syndrome occurring with some other
disease. Each case needs to be considered individually and only
examples of premenstrual syndrome should be included in
clinical trials. Thus premenstrual epilepsy, in which the electro-
encephalography and other investigations are normal, should be
included in premenstrual syndrome, but if the abnormal findings
persist during the postmenstruum it should not be included.
Some women with premenstrual asthma have unimpaired air

73

entry in the postmenstruum and come within the definition of premenstrual syndrome, while others have a premenstrual exacerbation of their asthma. The somatic symptoms discussed in this chapter can, on occasions, come within the definition of premenstrual syndrome.

Neurological system

Headaches

Most surveys show that after tension (with the three components of depression, irritability and lethargy), headache is the next commonest symptom of premenstrual syndrome (see Tables 5.2, 27.4, 27.5 & 27.18). (Dalton, 1954, 1973, 1982, Greene & Dalton, Kerr *et al.*, Watts *et al.*, Haspels *et al.*) Headaches are useful items to record on a menstrual chart when investigating the relationship of symptoms to menstruation. The patient often hesitates to record the symptoms of depression, irritability or lethargy, either because the onset is imperceptible or because she feels that the symptoms are evidence of her lack of self-control. The use of an attacks form (Fig. 3.12) is especially helpful when determining whether an individual attack of headache was provoked by relative hypoglycaemia or was due to a specific food such as cheese, chocolate or alcohol.

The premenstrual headaches are variable in character, ranging from dull, continuous, generalised ones, easily relieved by simple analgesics, to those preceded by visual or other aura and accompanied by prostration, vomiting and vertigo. Of premenstrual headaches, 60% tend to be centred on the eyes (Fig. 7.1) whereas occipital, vertical and temporal premenstrual headaches are rare (Greene & Dalton, 1953).

In 1975 a nationwide appeal by the British Migraine Association resulted in 886 non-pregnant women completing questionnaires together with a three-month record of their migraine attacks and menstruations. The survey covered 1239 menstruations and 936 migraine attacks. It proved possible to differentiate two types of migraine sufferers, those whose migraine appeared to be hormonally related and those with sporadic attacks (Dalton). The characteristics of the hormonally related group included the following:

1. Onset at puberty, after the contraceptive pill or after a pregnancy.

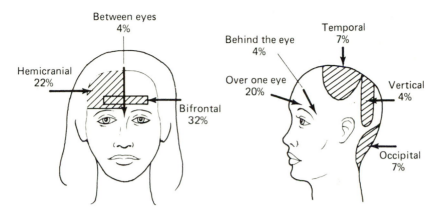

Fig. 7.1   Sites of pain in premenstrual headaches.

2. Attacks occurring at the same time in each menstrual cycle, viz. at ovulation or during the paramenstruum.
3. Freedom from attacks in late pregnancy.
4. Increase in severity of migraine after each pregnancy.
5. Deterioration of migraine on taking the contraceptive pill (only oestrogen-progestogen oral preparations were being used).
6. Improvement in severity and frequency of migraine two years after the menopause.

The time relationship of 512 headaches in sufferers of premenstrual migraine is shown in Fig. 7.2 (Dalton, 1973).

The marked relationship of menstruation in the 935 migraine attacks is shown in Fig. 7.3 in which the attacks are broken down among those 241 women currently on the pill, the 290 ex-takers and the 355 who had never taken the pill (Dalton, 1976).

Many known and unknown factors are responsible for headaches. Important trigger factors among those occurring predominantly during the paramenstruum appear to be relative hypoglycaemia, water retention, depression, and increased sensitivity to specific foods.

Epilepsy

Epilepsy is a culminating symptom of premenstrual syndrome, either as grand mal or, more rarely, as petit mal. The characteristics of premenstrual epilepsy are as follows:

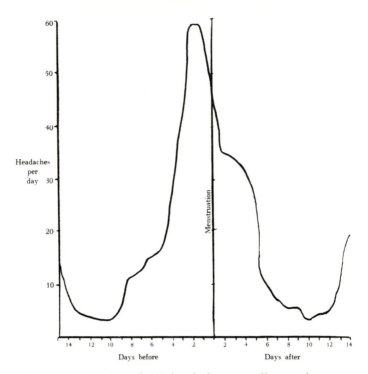

Fig. 7.2 Time relationship of 512 headaches in sufferers of premenstrual headache. (From Dalton K. (1973). *Headache*; **12:**4, 151.)

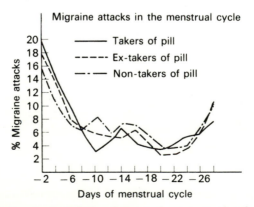

Fig. 7.3 Migraine attacks (935) in relation to the menstrual cycle. (From Dalton K. (1976), *Headache*; **15:**4, 247.)

1. Attacks limited to the paramenstruum.
2. Attacks preceded by tension and frequently a severe headache.
3. Onset of epilepsy coinciding with menarche, after a pregnancy (especially if complicated by pre-eclampsia), or while on oral contraceptives.
4. Freedom from attacks in late pregnancy.
5. Attacks occur after long intervals without food.

In a survey of 192 women who had previously suffered from pre-eclampsia it was noted that 10 women (5%) subsequently developed premenstrual grand mal (Dalton, 1954). This is a complication of pre-eclampsia which is too often overlooked. It is interesting that sufferers of premenstrual epilepsy frequently experience a severe headache before an attack that is similar to one experienced before an eclamptic fit (see Appendix and Table 27.19).

These patients can be controlled by progesterone therapy without the use of anticonvulsant drugs and because progesterone is not classified as an anticonvulsant, women suffering from premenstrual epilepsy controlled by progesterone may apply for a driving licence when they have been free from fits for two years. Progesterone also eliminates the dangers of short-term and long-term side effects of anticonvulsants. An incidence of 3% premenstrual epilepsy was noted in the survey reported in Table 5.2.

The charts of two women whose grand mal attacks were related to menstruation are shown in Fig. 7.4. In both cases there were also premenstrual symptoms of tension and headache, their attacks were precipitated by long intervals without food. Both obtained driving licences after three years' progesterone treatment and were able to stop anticonvulsants. The mother of two children had a short relapse five years later when she developed a large progesterone abscess in her buttocks and progesterone treatment was temporarily suspended.

Vertigo

Vertigo occurs in about a third of all sufferers, either accompanying a headache or occurring alone, and is aggravated by stooping. It is common in parous women approaching the menopause, and

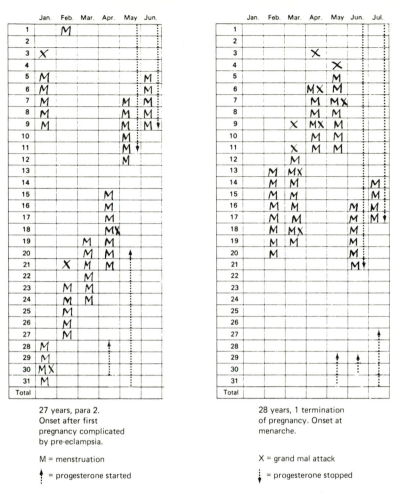

27 years, para 2.
Onset after first
pregnancy complicated
by pre-eclampsia.

28 years, 1 termination
of pregnancy. Onset at
menarche.

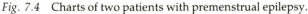

M = menstruation
↑ = progesterone started

X = grand mal attack
⋮ = progesterone stopped

Fig. 7.4 Charts of two patients with premenstrual epilepsy.

in those who have suffered from pre-eclampsia. It is probably due to increased fluid in the labyrinths (Table 27.5).

Syncope

Syncope is likely to occur after prolonged standing, such as queueing for lunch. There is usually a history of a long interval without food, probably after missing breakfast.

Paraesthesia

Paraesthesia of the hands and feet is common among those with water retention and symptoms of weight gain and bloatedness. In some patients the symptoms are initially limited to the para-menstruum and thus represent premenstrual syndrome, but later symptoms increase until they are present throughout the entire month, typical of the carpal tunnel syndrome; in such cases relief may be obtained by decompression of the median nerve. Paraesthesia is noted among those whose pregnancy has been complicated with pre-eclampsia or excessive weight gain. Occasionally the paraesthesia may represent the aura of a classical migraine attack.

Symptoms of the respiratory system

Asthma

Asthma occurred in 15% of the 610 women with premenstrual syndrome reported in Table 5.2 (see also Table 27.4 & 27.19).

Asthma often starts acutely in the middle of the night, continues for hours or days and then ends abruptly with the onset of menstruation. About a third of women of childbearing years attending asthma allergy clinics are noted to have a tendency to premenstrual attacks, especially around puberty and the meno-pause (Rees). The asthma is accompanied by tension, which is easily blamed on the distress caused by the asthma attack. When recording on a chart it is worth while noting the number of occasions that an aerosol inhaler is used for the relief of symptoms; only if inhalers are not required during the postmenstruum can the diagnosis of premenstrual syndrome be made (Hanley). Currently under the care of the premenstrual syndrome clinic at University College Hospital, London, are two women, aged 18 and 42 years who both had over 20 admissions to the intensive care unit for acute attacks of asthma before an alert ward sister recognised that their attacks were limited to the premenstruum. They have since been maintained on progesterone therapy and have required no further admissions.

Pneumothorax

There is an interesting report of a 41-year-old woman who had 25 recurrent attacks of right-sided spontaneous pneumothorax over a period of four years, always on the fourth day of menstruation. At thoracotomy, endometriosis of the diaphragm was found.

Otorhinolaryngological symptoms

Engorgement of the nasal mucous membrane occurring at menstruation is reputed to have been known by Hippocrates (Greene). It may result in nasal obstruction causing sinusitis or be misdiagnosed as a common cold. Recurrent colds in women of childbearing years should be regarded with suspicion and the time relationship of the attacks plotted against menstruation. The woman who complains in April that she has already had four colds since Christmas is always suspect – it may be a monthly occurrence related to menstruation.

Rhinitis

Rhinitis is another common cyclical allergic phenomenon – often referred to by laymen as the 'common cold' – which may be limited to the premenstruum.

Hoarseness

Hoarseness may occur during the premenstruum, and is especially noticed in opera singers. One opera singer arranged her engagements so that she avoided the paramenstruum. Another, who was treated with progesterone for the relief of premenstrual epilepsy, remarked that the quality of her voice and her ability to reach high notes had improved since starting treatment. The symptoms appear to be due to oedema of the vocal cords (Frable).

Diminution of the sense of smell

The loss of the sense of smell is common. The manufacturers of a deodorant/antiperspirant noticed that women changed their brand after three or four weeks' use, complaining that it had ceased to function effectively. It was then realised that the women's dissatisfaction was due to a premenstrual increase in sweating and vaginal discharge and a diminishing perception of the reassuring perfume of the deodorant/antiperspirant product. This had led women falsely to conclude that the product had lost its efficiency.

Gastrointestinal symptoms

Abdominal bloatedness occurred in 33% of 1095 women (Table 27.5), and causes considerable embarrassment to those of slim build who have to change into loose-fitting clothes. An increase in girth of 5–10cm may be tolerated without complaint by the obese, but not by the figure-conscious. It is best measured at the level of the umbilicus when lying down and when standing, at different phases of the cycle. The standing measurement increases premenstrually. If there is no apparent difference in measurement in relation to menstruation it is more likely to be due to laxity of the anterior abdominal wall. Some women complain of heaviness and dragging pains associated with the bloatedness, which is a symptom of water retention. There is not necessarily any relation between the intensity of the bloatedness and the change in weight.

Food cravings and compulsive eating are frequently reported by sufferers from premenstrual syndrome, especially among those on strict weight-reducing diets, who find they can maintain their permitted food intake during the postmenstrual and preovulatory phases but during the premenstruum they gorge chocolates, sweets and high carbohydrate foods in large quantities. A slim typist described how she crept downstairs after midnight to eat two whole loaves of bread when previously she had limited herself to one slice daily (see Table 27.5).

Smith and Sauder noted in a questionnaire survey to 300 nurses that food cravings were positively related to premenstrual depression and water retention. It is perhaps comforting to know that female rhesus monkeys reject their food around ovulation, but regain their appetite during the premenstruum. Czaja (1975) showed that in 46 female rhesus monkeys, in 112 cycles, this food rejection at ovulation was related to the oestrogen level (Fig. 7.5).

Nausea and Vomiting may occur as accompanying symptoms of headache or bloatedness, but they rarely occur alone.

Constipation is a common premenstrual symptom related to water retention. By contrast, diarrhoea is an uncommon symptom except in those suffering from ulcerative colitis, who may notice a premenstrual deterioration. If a woman claims a link between diarrhoea and menstruation it is important to investigate thoroughly and arrange careful charting. On more than one occasion intermittent diarrhoea has been found to be due to Sonne dysentery.

Urinary symptoms

Oliguria is accompanied by oedema and weight gain during the premenstruum and followed by a spontaneous diuresis during

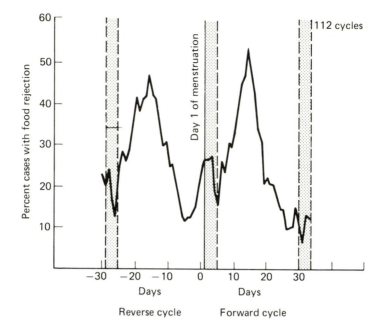

Fig. 7.5 Changes in food rejection during the Rhesus female menstrual cycle. Shaded area=mean menses interval. (From Czaja J. (1975). *Physiology and Behaviour*; **14**:582.)

menstruation. As in idiopathic oedema it may be accompanied by nocturnal frequency with increased urinary excretion occurring in association with the horizontal posture.

Urethritis and *Cystitis* commonly recur during the premenstruum and may be due to the increase in vaginal discharge or to retention cysts in the urethra. In the absence of infection, progesterone treatment is most effective.

Enuresis is a troublesome symptom in an adult, but when limited to the premenstruum is amenable to treatment. It occurs in those who were late to develop bladder control in childhood and may be accompanied by hypersomnia. It occurred in 1% of women with premenstrual syndrome reported in the Appendix (Table 27.5.)

Urinary retention is rarely seen during the paramenstruum, and appears to result from oedema of the urinary sphincter. A 17-year-old boarding school girl was admitted to hospital on eight occasions for premenstrual urinary retention. Full renal investigations were normal, and then it was noted that the dates of hospital admissions were correlated with the dates of menstruation. She was successfully treated with progesterone.

Symptoms of the musculoskeletal system

Joint and muscle pains may be noted only during the pre-menstruum, especially when there is a history of injury, and characteristically there is increased pain and stiffness on waking. Pains may be present for a few days in the back, hip, knees, ankles, shoulders, hands and feet and then miraculously vanish only to reappear with the next premenstruum. The pain may be due to localised oedema or to failure of muscle relaxation. The most likely candidates are parous women over 35 years. Figure 7.6 shows sites of premenstrual joint and muscle pains.

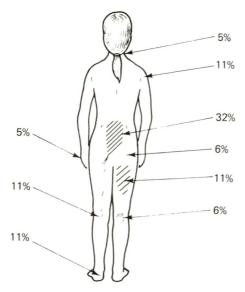

Fig. 7.6   Sites of premenstrual joint and muscle pains.

Breast symptoms

Breast enlargement, with pain and tenderness of the nipples, tends to start at ovulation and increases in severity until the onset of menstruation. Transient masses or cysts may occur in the breast premenstrually; these disappear spontaneously or decrease in size during menstruation. It is akin to the breast activity occurring early in pregnancy. Breasts should always be examined for galactorrhoea and, if present, the prolactin level should be estimated. Breast tenderness was present in 22% of 1095 women (Table 27.5).

Cardiovascular symptoms

Palpitations, Ectopic beats and *Paroxysmal tachycardia* are all symptoms which have been reported to recur during the premenstruum. These symptoms call for a full cardiological investigation as well as the recording of symptoms in relation to menstruation. There may be accompanying dyspnoea, weight gain and oedema.

Dermatological symptoms

Boils, Acne and *Herpes Zoster* are common premenstrual symptoms. Most skin disorders have a cyclical variation in relation to menstruation, but if the underlying pathological process continues throughout the cycle they should not be considered premenstrual syndrome.
Facial pigmentation waxes and wanes with each menstruation due to increasing secretion of melanocyte-stimulating hormone of the pituitary.
Urticaria may recur as an allergic reaction in the premenstruum but the allergen is unknown.

Eye symptoms

Conjunctivitis of the non-infective type may occur either unilaterally or bilaterally, and presents as a red, watery, irritable eye. Its relationship to the menstrual cycle was noted as early as the sixteenth century (Ray). It may be accompanied by sneezing, and may be related to the premenstrual engorgement of the nasal mucous membrane causing reflex stimulation of the fifth cranial nerve (Glass).
Styes are another common recurrent symptom related to the lowered resistance to infection during the paramenstruum.
Glaucoma: premenstrual syndrome and closed angle glaucoma

have many points of similarity. Thus both: (1) can be provoked by the water drinking test; (2) are more severe in the early morning; (3) are increased or precipitated by stress and fatigue; and (4) are accompanied by other systemic disturbances such as nausea, lethargy and vertigo.

In a survey at the Institute of Ophthalmology, London, 89% of sufferers of closed-angle glaucoma also had premenstrual syndrome, compared with only 50% among those with simple chronic glaucoma (Dalton, 1967). Again, there was a high incidence (21%) of pre-eclampsia among the parous sufferers of all types of glaucoma. The timing of 356 episodes of ocular symptoms in 106 menstrual cycles showed 49% occurred during the paramenstruum. The influence of menstruation on the timing of ocular symptoms was almost entirely confined to the closed-angle glaucoma with 60% occurring during the paramenstruum (Fig. 7.7) compared with 30% among those with simple chronic glaucoma (Fig. 7.8).

Regular observations have shown a pattern of raised intra-ocular pressure with a simultaneous rise in blood pressure and weight during the paramenstruum. Each patient has her own timing of the rise, some showing a rise in the premenstruum

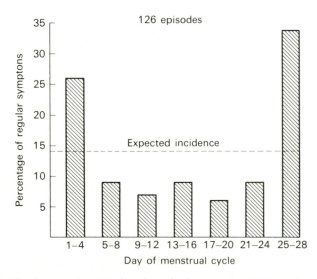

Fig. 7.7 Ocular symptoms in closed-angle glaucoma in relation to the menstrual cycle. (From Dalton K. (1967). *Br. J. Ophthal.*; **51**:10, 692.)

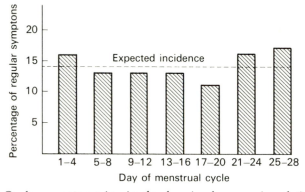

Fig. 7.8 Ocular symptoms in simple chronic glaucoma in relation to the menstrual cycle. (From Dalton K. (1967). *Br. J. Ophthal.*; **51**:10, 692.)

followed by a drop during menstruation before returning to the intermenstrual level, and other women showing a premenstrual drop followed by a pronounced menstrual rise before returning to normality (Fig. 7.9). This is related to the time of the full menstrual flow, as discussed on p. 48 and Fig 5.1.

Contact lenses become a problem among sufferers of the premenstrual syndrome, who should be advised to have all the fittings and to begin wearing them during the postmenstruum. One frequently hears the remark after progesterone treatment, 'Now I can wear my contact lenses all the month round'.

Conjunctival and *Retinal haemorrhages* may result from premenstrual capillary fragility.

Behcet's Syndrome with its triad of relapsing iridocyclitis and associated recurrent ulceration of the mouth and genitalia has been noted to have a periodicity coincident with menstruation but the pathological process continues throughout the cycle and it should not be considered premenstrual syndrome (Hutfield).

Uveitis tends to have recurrence during the paramenstruum but again the pathological process continues throughout the cycle.

Dental symptoms

Ulcerative stomatitis and *Buccal ulceration* occurring during the premenstruum may be independent or may occur coincidentally with ulceration of the vulva, lower vagina or anus; in some cases it may be due to recurrent herpes.

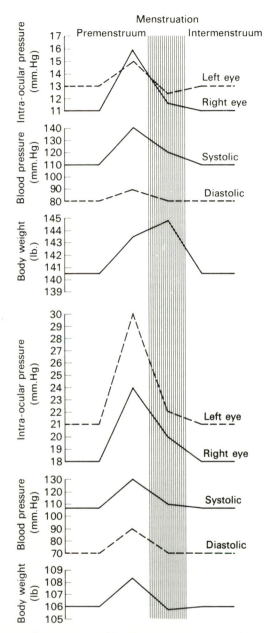

Fig. 7.9 Intraocular pressure, blood pressure and weight in patients with closed-angle glaucoma. (From Dalton K. (1967). *Br. J. Ophthal.*; **51**:10, 692.)

Drug reactions

These are common during the premenstruum and may follow administration of antibiotics and inoculations. Confusion may occur as to the real origin of such reactions. In double-blind clinical trials the placebo drugs are often reported to have side effects such as increased drowsiness, headache, nausea, or increased pain, which may be no more than the usual premenstrual symptoms which have been scrupulously observed and reported.

Cosmetic symptoms

During the premenstruum the woman may be conscious of not looking her best due to a puffy face, thick lips, dark shadows under her eyes, the presence of acne and pimples, and lank, greasy hair.

Signs

Oedema of the ankles (especially in women whose work includes prolonged standing), *abdomen and fingers* is common, but does not occur in all patients. It may be noticed by the patient when her shoes will not tie up, her wedding ring becomes too tight, her dresses no longer fit comfortably, she develops facial pallor, or her dentures no longer fit because of swollen gums. Characteristically, oedema increases in hot weather. When oedema is already present, as in congenital lymphatic oedema or lymphatic obstruction after radical mastectomy, there may be a further increase during the premenstruum.

Fluctuations of blood pressure throughout the menstrual cycle are frequent, with rises of 20 to 30mmHg during the premenstruum when symptoms are present. Rises from 110/70 to 140/90mmHg may occur, but rarely does blood pressure rise to hypertensive levels. On the other hand, hypotension may occur when the onset of an attack is sudden and accompanied by pronounced oedema. A severe case of premenstrual cyclical oedema has been described in which a 34-year-old woman sometimes gained as much as 5kg in less than 24 hours, these episodes being accompanied by severe shock and hypotension (Clarkson).

Proteinuria may occasionally occur in severe cases during the premenstruum, especially in those prone to epilepsy. For its detection it is necessary to use either catheter specimens or carefully collected midstream specimens, because slight menstrual staining may otherwise contaminate the urine.

Fig. 7.10 shows observations on a 40-year-old housewife with no children, who was suffering from premenstrual headaches, depression and irritability. There was a rise in blood pressure from 110/70mmHg after menstruation to 140–160/80mmHg in the premenstruum, and the proteinuria in catheter specimens was limited to the premenstruum. Treatment with progesterone brought relief of all symptoms; the blood pressure did not rise and there was no proteinuria.

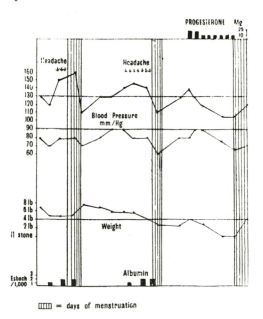

IIIII = days of menstruation

Fig. 7.10   Blood pressure, weight and albumin in patient with premenstrual syndrome.

Fig. 7.11 shows observations on a 42-year-old housewife with no children, who was suffering from premenstrual headache, depression, oedema and dyspnoea. It shows a weight gain of 5kg in a 44.5kg woman, this weight being lost by diuresis during menstruation. Proteinuria was present in the premenstruum and early morning measurements of the ankle circumference showed an increase of 18.4cm to 24.6cm. At the height of the oedema moist sounds were present in the bases of both lungs, accounting no

doubt for the dyspnoea. The blood pressure was raised throughout the cycle at a level of 200–250/121–130mmHg: this is therefore
an example of hypertension with premenstrual exacerbation of
symptoms and not premenstrual syndrome. On treatment with
progesterone she became symptom-free, her weight and ankle
circumference remained steady, and there was no proteinuria.
Nevertheless, the hypertension persisted at its previous high
level throughout the cycle.

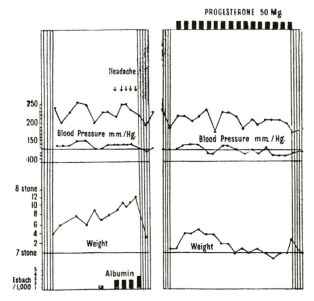

Fig. 7.11   Blood pressure, weight and albumin in patient with essential
hypertension.

Fig. 7.12 shows observations on a 40-year-old club hostess, who
had been unemployed for six months because of premenstrual
epileptic fits and migraine. She was a widow whose only
pregnancy had been terminated at 28 weeks because of chronic
nephritis. Immediately before a premenstrual epileptic fit she
had a blood pressure of 190/110mmHg which dropped to
120–130/80mmHg after menstruation. Premenstrually her weight
rose by 0.9kg and the ankle circumference increased from 19cm to
22cm. The proteinuria was present throughout the cycle and so
this is again an example of premenstrual exacerbation of nephritis

and is not premenstrual syndrome. When treated with progesterone she became symptom-free, blood pressure, weight and ankle circumference becoming steady, but the proteinuria persisted throughout the cycle. No epileptic fits have occurred since starting progesterone 20 years ago.

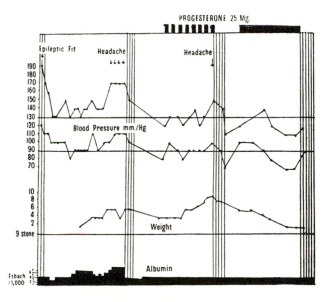

Fig. 7.12   Blood pressure, weight and albumin in patient with chronic nephritis.

Spontaneous bruising may occur because of increased capillary fragility during the premenstruum (Billig & Spaulding). The bruises are painless, bilateral, usually all about the same size and circular. Common sites are the thighs and upper arms. One such spontaneous bruise was observed developing on the upper arm while at rest and spread from a sudden red dot to a bruise which reached a diameter of 2.6cm. It was quite painless and the time from first noticing it to its completion took barely a minute. Hess's test (with 80mmHg for 10 minutes) may be used to test capillary fragility in women and an increase during premenstruum, rising to a maximum around the first day of menstruation, may be noted. There are considerable individual variations in maximal fragilities. European women tend to have higher fragilities than Chinese or Malaysian women.

8

Incidence

Premenstrual syndrome is 'the presence of recurrent symptoms in the premenstruum with the absence of symptoms in the postmenstruum'.

Premenstrual syndrome has been described as 'one of the world's commonest diseases', but the true incidence is difficult to assess and is dependent on the definition used in the survey (see Chapter 2). The diagnosis of the premenstrual syndrome with the many, varied somatic and psychological symptoms depends partly on the intelligence of the patient and partly on her medical adviser. It is likely that as members of the public become increasingly better educated by the media on menstrual problems the incidence of premenstrual syndrome may appear to increase.

Another aspect of the problem is that in some of the surveys, women suffering from recognised somatic symptoms have been deliberately excluded as when 'all those on regular medication' or 'suffering from organic disease' are not included in the population studies. Other surveys are carried out in factories which do not employ epileptics, or among university students with above-average intelligence. In yet other surveys, usually by psychologists, a menstrual distress questionnaire is used, emphasising the psychological symptoms. The incidence of the premenstrual syndrome depends on the criteria adopted. Thus Pennington found an incidence of 95% while Logan and Cushion found it to be 6.5% in their general practice. Neither of these figures is likely to be correct. Kessel and Coppen in a survey into the menstrual problems of 500 English women, chosen at random from ten general practitioners' lists, concluded that the incidence was very high and that there were two common but distinct entities – the premenstrual syndrome and dysmenorrhoea.

In 1954, a survey of 825 women in north London limited premenstrual syndrome to: 'Those whose premenstrual symptoms have been present for three menstrual cycles as confirmed by a prospective calendar, and with symptoms severe enough to demand medical attention or loss of work in the past three months.' The incidence was found to be 27% for controls and 86% among women who had previously suffered from pre-eclampsia (Dalton, 1954). If one uses less strict criteria, to include symptoms endured or self-treated and not confirming the relationship to menstruation with a calendar, an incidence of 40% may be expected in the general population in Britain (Fig. 8.1).

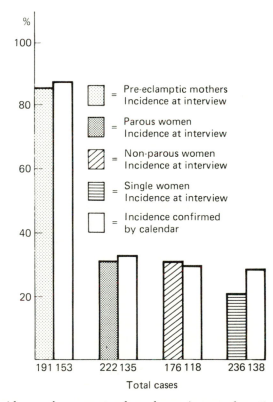

Fig. 8.1 Incidence of premenstrual syndrome in pre-eclamptic mothers and normal women. (From Dalton K. (1964). (*Premenstrual Syndrome*; Fig.12, p.40.)

More surveys are needed in specialty clinics for example, asthma, obesity, epilepsy, cardiac, infertility, colitis, hypertension or otitis clinics – to determine the proportion of women who have exacerbations of their distress at the time of menstruation, and those whose symptoms are present only in the paramenstruum.

Age and parity

The age (Tables 8.1 & 27.2) and parity (Tables 8.2 & 27.3) distribution of 610 and of 1095 women seen in 1982, who had been referred by their general practitioners for severe premenstrual syndrome, suggests that although premenstrual syndrome frequently starts at puberty it does not become a serious problem until after the age of 30 years (Dalton, 1982).

Lloyd emphasised the fact that hitherto unaffected women often begin to experience the premenstrual syndrome in their fourth decade and suggested the designation 'mid-thirties syndrome' although this is not to imply that the condition differs substantially from that of women in other age groups.

Parity tends to increase with age and premenstrual symptoms increase with parity. It is interesting that of 457 women who had been pregnant only 18 (4%) had not succeeded in having a full-term pregnancy (Table 8.2). The abortions included both spontaneous and therapeutic ones, so it is difficult to draw conclusions (see also Table 27.3).

Not all sufferers have an easy conception, for Benedek-Jaszmann and Hearn-Sturtevant studied 45 patients with pre-

Table 8.1

Age on starting progesterone

Years	n=610 n	%
Under 20	29	5
„ 25	43	7
„ 30	75	12
„ 35	182	30
„ 40	131	21
„ 45	79	13
„ 50	47	8
Over 50	25	4

Table 8.2

Parity at first consultation

	n=610
No pregnancies	153
No full-term pregnancies	18
One full-term pregnancies	129
Two full-term pregnancies	207
Three full-term pregnancies	81
Four or more full-term pregnancies	22
No abortions	277
One abortion	122
Two abortions	32
Three abortions	11
Four or more abortions	15

menstrual syndrome who were attending an infertility clinic in the Netherlands.

Pre-eclampsia

It has already been mentioned that 86% of women who have had a pregnancy complicated by pre-enclampsia subsequently developed premenstrual symptoms (Fig. 8.1) (Dalton, 1954). Of the 100 consecutive hospital patients, 75 had full-term pregnancies and 15 (20%) suffered from pre-eclampsia. This is a similar finding to that of Greene and Dalton in 1953 who reported that in 58 parous women with premenstrual syndrome 11 (19%) gave a history of pre-eclampsia. It was this finding which led to the survey into the incidence of premenstrual syndrome in women who had previously suffered a pre-eclamptic pregnancy and led, ultimately, to the appreciation of the similarity of these two diseases (Chapter 20) (see also Table 27.11).

There are several patients with the premenstrual syndrome under my care in whose case history there is a note that their mother had an eclamptic fit during the patient's birth, but the exact incidence of premenstrual syndrome among those whose mothers had eclampsia at their birth is not yet known.

Postnatal depression

In the survey of 610 women with premenstrual syndrome, a high incidence of postnatal depression – 56% – was noted (Dalton, 1982). Some of these women dated the onset of premenstrual syndrome as following the postnatal depression, while others reported that the syndrome had been present before the pregnancy but that the severity of premenstrual symptoms had increased after postnatal depression eased (Table 8.3) (see also Table 27.11).

Table 8.3

History at first visit of women with premenstrual syndrome

| | *(n=439 with full-term pregnancies)* | |
	n	%
Pre-eclampsia	59	13
Postnatal depression	254	58
Sterilisation	62	14

Familial incidence

A mother who suffers from the premenstrual syndrome may find that her daughter suffers from the same symptoms as herself and she is most likely to recognise and diagnose it in her daughter at adolescence. But the mother who suffered from spasmodic dysmenorrhoea in her youth is often surprised when her daughter develops similar symptoms after having two or three years of pain-free menstruation. There does appear to be a genetic link in premenstrual syndrome. Kantero and Widholm's study of premenstrual symptoms occurring in adolescent daughters and their mothers revealed that 63% of daughters of symptom-free mothers were also symptom-free. If the mother had premenstrual fatigue or irritability, nearly 70% of daughters had similar symptoms. Adopted daughters tend to have the same type of menstruation as their natural mothers, be it spasmodic dysmenorrhoea or premenstrual syndrome, rather than that of their adoptive mothers, suggesting that it is not a learnt pattern. Similarly, among identical twins the same type of menstruation is present, in contrast with unidentical twins, who show an incidence of premenstrual syndrome as would be expected on a chance distribution.

While recognising the wide range of possible symptoms there is a tendency for members of the same family to present with similar symptoms. Thus some families are troubled most with depression, and others by migraine, asthma or epilepsy. If one member of the family presents with a good record showing correlation of symptoms with the menstrual cycle, and the next member gives a history of similar symptoms but without any record of time relationship to the menstrual cycle there is a strong possibility that the next month's recording will confirm the diagnosis of premenstrual syndrome. Indeed there are occasions on which, if there is a strong family history it would be justifiable to begin treatment before a positive record is available. Several members of three or four generations have been seen who all have the same manifestation, which may not be surprising as migraine and allergic phenomenon are frequently familial manifestations.

Cultural variations

Janiger and his colleagues have done an interesting study in which they administered a simple questionnaire of 32 symptoms followed by the four words 'no', 'mild', 'moderate' and 'severe' to 479 women of different cultures and asked them to describe the intensity of each symptom in the week before the most recent menstruation. Premenstrual symptoms were found in all cultures, although several showed symptom variations between the culture groups. The most outstanding was the paucity of breast complaints in the Japanese, which may be related to their low incidence of breast cancer (Fig. 8.2).

The high incidence of headaches among the Nigerians was notable (Fig. 8.3). The mean premenstrual symptom scores were highest among the Turkish and lowest among the Japanese. To the question of which was the most distressing premenstrual symptom the answer in all culture groups was lower abdominal pain. The authors concluded that the study did not support the hypothesis that premenstrual symptoms follow the degree of comfort and complexity of today's living.

Post-hysterectomy and post-oophorectomy symptoms

Cyclical symptoms, of the same type as the individual's previous premenstrual symptoms, may occur after hysterectomy, bilateral oophorectomy, or artificial menopause by radiotherapy, although there is usually an interval of 6–12 months before the symptoms resume their full severity (Chapter 23) (Dalton, 1957). In one series of 34 women who had hysterectomies for non-

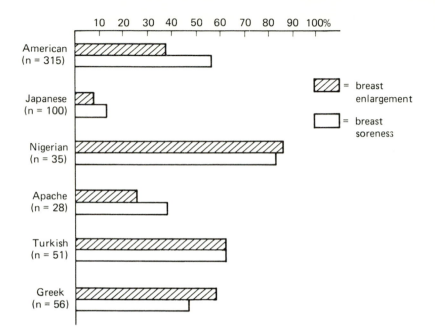

Fig. 8.2   Incidence in ethnic groups of premenstrual breast enlargement and
soreness. (Compiled from Janiger O. *et al.* (1972). *Psychosomatics*;
13:226–35.)

malignant conditions, as many as 74% had cyclically recurrent
headaches. In half of these women the headaches had in fact
occurred premenstrually before operative intervention, but the
headaches increased in intensity after hysterectomy, often
accompanied by vomiting, photophobia and blurred vision
(Dalton, 1957). In the survey of 610 women with premenstrual
syndrome reported in Table 8.4, 8% had a hysterectomy and 3% a
bilateral oophorectomy (see also Table 27.24).

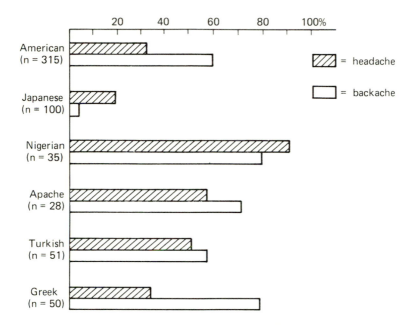

Fig. 8.3 Incidence in ethnic groups of premenstrual headaches and backaches.
(Compiled from Janiger O. *et al.* (1972). *Psychosomatics;* **13**:226–35.)

Table 8.4

Conditions at first visit of 610 women with premenstrual syndrome

	n=610	
	n	%
Premenstrual syndrome	504	83
Hysterectomy/oophorectomy	68	11
Postnatal depression	26	4
Pregnant	9	1
Others	3	1

9

Aetiology

Premenstrual syndrome is 'the presence of recurrent symptoms in the premenstruum with absence of symptoms in the postmenstruum'.

The many hormonal interactions which result in premenstrual syndrome are not fully understood. Numerous theories and conflicting evidence confuse the casual reader on premenstrual syndrome. The definition should be clearly stated (Chapter 1) as should the method by which the diagnosis has been made (Chapter 2). A premenstrual exacerbation of an underlying disease is not premenstrual syndrome. The many problems associated with research and clinical trials of premenstrual syndrome are discussed in Chapter 17.

One must *not* accept the patient's word that she has premenstrual syndrome, experience in premenstrual syndrome clinics suggests that only between 18% and 30% of patients have the diagnosis confirmed. Premenstrual syndrome must surely be one of the few diseases that is persistently being investigated in patients who do *not* have the disease. In a survey carried out in a clinic where the author once worked, 85 patients were referred with premenstrual syndrome, but after careful history-taking, examination and some hormonal investigations, 55 women were shown to be suffering from some other illness – for example, hypothyroidism, hyperprolactinaemia, depression, constipation, polycystic ovaries. The remaining 30 women gave clear histories of premenstrual syndrome, but on charting their symptoms only 15 (18%) were found to have premenstrual syndrome; the remaining 15 women had symptoms in the postmenstruum and premenstruum. The patients were given a placebo while charting their symptoms, and seven of the women without premenstrual syndrome responded to the placebo, but none of the correctly diagnosed patients with premenstrual syndrome benefited from the placebo.

When considering explanations of the hormonal imbalance that results in premenstrual syndrome the obvious starting point is the normal menstrual cycle, for premenstrual syndrome is a disease with symptoms limited to the last 14 days of the cycle. This is also the time when progesterone is in greatest concentration in the peripheral blood. Early workers measured urinary pregnandiol, which is the metabolic excretion product of progesterone, and noted a low level of urinary pregnandiol in sufferers of premenstrual syndrome. More recently workers have measured plasma progesterone levels by radioimmunoassays and found it low in some sufferers of premenstrual syndrome, when compared with controls (Backstrom and Cartenson, 1974, and Munday, 1977) (Fig. 9.1). Moreover, the plasma progesterone

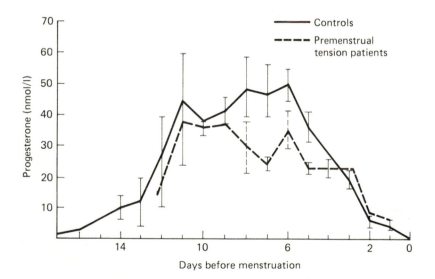

Note: days dated backwards from 1st day of menstruation

Fig. 9.1   Mean plasma progesterone values in eight controls and in eight women with premenstrual syndrome. Note: days dated backwards from first day of menstruation. (From Munday M.R. *et al.* (1981). *Clin. Endocrin;* **14**:1–9.)

concentration in those with premenstrual syndrome was higher than in women who do not ovulate, although it is clear that not every woman who does not ovulate suffers from premenstrual syndrome. Thus, the low plasma progesterone level in the luteal phase found in premenstrual syndrome patients is not the full answer. Both groups of workers also found, in premenstrual syndrome patients, a slightly higher plasma oestradiol level at the end of the luteal phase when compared with controls.

Both progesterone and oestradiol are bound in the plasma to specific binding proteins and to non-specific binding proteins such as albumin (Speroff *et al.*). The free unbound steroid is the biologically active fraction. Progesterone is bound to cortisol binding globulin (CBG, previously called transcortin) which also binds cortisol. Careful control is needed to maintain free cortisol levels within the desired range in the body and therefore one would not expect to find major alterations in the cortisol binding globulin levels in patients with premenstrual syndrome because they would then also show changes in cortisol metabolism.

Oestradiol is bound to sex hormone binding globulin (SHBG) which also binds testosterone and, to an even higher affinity, dihydrotestosterone. Changes in SHBG levels alter oestradiol and testosterone levels and, as testosterone binds to SHBG with a greater affinity, changes in SHBG levels reflect greater changes in oestradiol levels.

The SHBG levels, measured by Iqbal and Johnson's two tier method, in 50 women with severe premenstrual syndrome and 50 controls showed significantly lower SHBG levels in the women with premenstrual syndrome (Fig. 3.10) (Dalton M. E., 1982). Low SHBG results in a higher free oestradiol in premenstrual syndrome women. Administration of progesterone raises the low SHBG in women with severe premenstrual syndrome (Dalton M. E., 1984).

During the second half of the luteal phase in a normal menstrual cycle many follicles in the ovary under the influence of oestradiol begin to lay down follicle stimulating hormone receptors (FSH receptors). When an FSH receptor has been filled by an FSH molecule it becomes the key that switches on the production of further oestradiol. This increased oestradiol production stimulates more FSH receptors to receive still more FSH. Thus, in the normal cycle one follicle produces more FSH receptors than the rest and develops a higher concentration of oestradiol, in this manner the Graafian follicle of that cycle develops while the other follicles gradually become atretic. The winning follicle is apparent by the middle of the follicular phase. In this follicle, in the presence of oestradiol, FSH promotes the production of the luteinising hormone receptors (LH receptors) which in turn bind to LH from the hypothalamus enabling the follicle to produce progesterone once it becomes a corpus luteum in the luteal phase.

The following hypothesis is proposed to explain, at the ovarian level, the findings in premenstrual syndrome patients with low progesterone levels and raised oestradiol level in the late luteal phase and raised FSH in the follicular phase (Bäckström; Cartenson; Munday et al.). The increased free oestradiol at the end of the luteal phase allows more than the usual number of follicles to develop. This increased number of follicles develops more FSH receptors spreading the uptake of FSH over still more follicles, with the result that the follicle which goes on to mature in that cycle has relatively fewer FSH receptors than would have been the case if fewer follicles had been stimulated to develop FSH receptors. As it has fewer FSH receptors it will bind to less FSH, which will be reflected in fewer LH receptors and less intrafollicular LH to stimulate progesterone production. This would result in lower progesterone production and more oestradiol in the late luteal phase, in this manner a self-perpetuating cycle would develop.

The gonadotrophins FHS and LH are secreted by the pituitary, together with prolactin. Prolactin has been considered an aetiological factor in premenstrual syndrome (Horrobin; Benedek-Jaszmann & Hearn-Sturtevant; Jeske et al. & Halbreich), but normal prolactin levels have been found by Bäckström and Aakvaag. Prolactin is a stress hormone and many women are extremely stressed in the luteal phase if they have premenstrual syndrome, so it is difficult to exclude the possibility that the raised prolactin concentrations sometimes found in premenstrual syndrome are the effect and not the cause. The levels of prolactin reported have never been very high and, as it is known that the normal distribution of prolactin is a log-skew distribution, the significance of these marginally raised values is difficult to interpret. It is known that increased prolactin levels interfere with steroidogenesis; however, severe hyperprolactinaemia usually results in a hypo-oestrogenised amenorrhoeric female, whereas patients with premenstrual syndrome have increased oestradiol levels (Munday et al.).

There is no evidence to suggest that aldosterone concentration significantly differs in patients with premenstrual syndrome compared with controls (Munday *et al.*).

While the pituitary secretes FSH and LH, which in turn influence oestradiol and progesterone production, it is the hypothalamus which controls the pituitary secretion of these gonadotrophins. Just as our knowledge of the role of FSH, LH and steroid production by the ovary during the menstrual cycle has increased, so too has our understanding of the hypothalamus. It is now recognised that the hypothalamus is a collection of areas which interact one with another to control gonadotrophin release among its other functions. The hypothalamus is situated near the floor of the third ventricle and special cells, known as 'tancytes' have been found that have ciliated cell bodies lining the floor of the third ventricle and ending in the portal system of the hypo-thalmus (Speroff *et al.*). Thus substances found in the cerebro-spinal fluid, such as steroids, endorphins and pineal gland secretions, will all affect the gonadotrophin release. There have been suggestions recently that endorphins or alpha-melanocyte stimulating hormone (α MSH) secretion may moderate the mood and behaviour changes of premenstrual syndrome (Reid and Yen).

A more realistic view may be to state that the control of the hormonal changes of the menstrual cycle is complex and influenced at various different levels by numerous hormonal and neurological events and the fault, therefore, may lie anywhere along the pathway from the cerebral cortex, along the hypothala-mic-pituitary-ovarian axis to the progesterone receptors in the tissue cells, but it appears that the progesterone transport mechanism (SHBG) is involved in all cases of severe premen-strual syndrome.

Progesterone is a basic building-block steroid from which many other steroids can be synthesised, it is so ubiquitous that, if given in sufficient doses, it could correct the resultant effects even if the lowered progesterone level were not the direct cause. For example, progesterone is known to decrease brain activity (Bäckström) and to have anticonvulsant properties (Merryman *et al.*, Spiegel *et al.*, Costa and Bonnycastle), hence its effectiveness in premenstrual epilepsy. By influencing the insulin receptors on the monocytes it will affect glucose metabolism and relieve the symptoms of transient hypoglycaemia. The immunosuppressive effect will reduce the incidence of infection and allergic reactions (Sitteri *et al.*).

More work must be done before we can establish beyond doubt the cause of premenstrual syndrome, but there is sufficient evidence to assure us that it is a hormonal illness and not a psychological one.

In some respects we can compare it with diabetes, which has many causes, the mild cases of which may be managed by dietary restriction but in severe cases, from whatever cause, treatment has to be with insulin. Similarly in premenstrual syndrome, with our present knowledge, progesterone is the treatment of choice in severe cases regardless of its aetiology.

10

The differences between progesterone and progestogens

Premenstrual syndrome is 'the presence of recurrent symptoms in the premenstruum with absence of symptoms in the postmenstruum'.

The basic steroid ring structure has played a vital part in the biochemical evolution of plants and animals. Relatively small changes in the degree of unsaturation and the number and nature of substituents have a striking influence on the biochemical activity of compounds such as are shown in Fig. 10.1. It is therefore not surprising that superficially similar synthetic derivatives have different actions from natural hormones.

Progesterone

The corpus luteum hormone was first isolated by Corner and Allen in 1929, and given the name progesterone by the Special Conference of the Health Organisation of the League of Nations in 1935.

Progesterone is secreted in the corpus luteum and passes from the ovary to the endometrium in increasing amounts from the time of ovulation. It reaches a peak of about 15μg/ml in the plasma about Day 21 to 23 and then the level falls until the onset of menstruation. Consequently the time of premenstrual symptoms coincides with the presence of progesterone in the blood (Fig. 10.2).

During pregnancy, progesterone is secreted from the ovary in

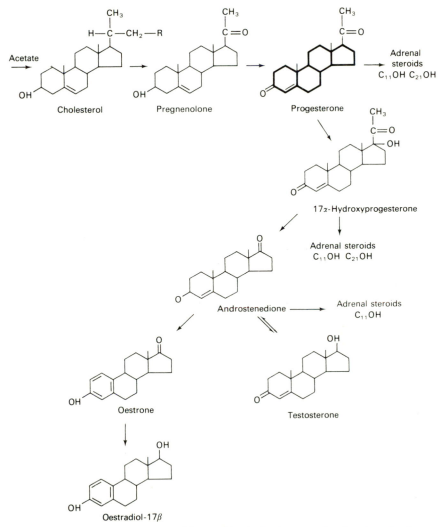

Fig. 10.1   Pathways in steroid biosynthesis in the gonads showing the key
position of progesterone. (From *Hormonal Assays and their Clinical
Applications* (1971). Loraine J.A., Bell E.T.E., Livingstone, S.)

increasing amounts for the first three months. The secretion of
progesterone from the placenta starts about the 9th week and is
then secreted in increasing amounts until the 32nd week, when
it probably remains steady until term and reaches a mean of
150 µg/ml plasma (Fig. 10.3).

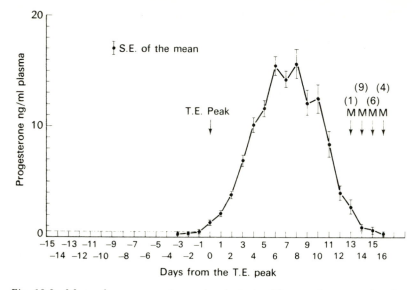

Fig. 10.2   Mean plasma progesterone levels during 20 normal menstrual cycles. (From Johansson E.D.B. (1969). *Acta Endocrin.* Copenhagen; **61**:592.)

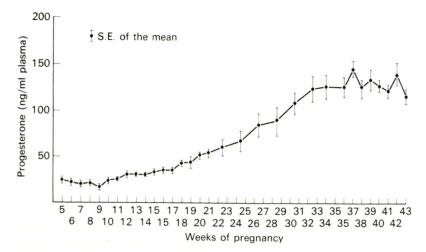

Fig. 10.3   Mean plasma progesterone during pregnancy. (From Johansson E.D.B. (1969), *Acta Endocrin.* Copenhagen; **61**:607.)

The functions of progesterone are to promote the following:

1. The development of the endometrium.
2. The maintenance of pregnancy.
3. The development of breast tissue.
4. The synthesis of corticosteroids in the adrenal cortex.
5. Lowering of the glucose tolerance.
6. Immunosuppression.
7. Action as an anticonvulsant.

The action of progesterone is species-specific, for instance, in man it reduces water and sodium retention (Landau *et al.*), but in dogs progesterone causes water retention (Thorne & Engel).

Progesterone is derived from cholesterol and is essential for the synthesis of a large number of steroid hormones, including the corticosteroids, the androgens and the oestrogens (Fig. 10.1).

The major metabolite of progesterone is pregnanediol, which can be isolated quantitatively in a 24-hour urine collection. Varying proportions of the metabolites are excreted in the urine, via the bile in the faeces, in the expired air and the skin.

Progesterone has a short half-life in the blood of only a few minutes and is relatively ineffective when given by mouth because it passes via the portal system to the liver where it is rapidly metabolised; however, it can be administered by intramuscular injections, or rectally or vaginally, or by implantation into the fat of the abdominal wall. Nillius and Johansson have suggested that when given by injection progesterone is absorbed into the fat cells where it forms a depot, and diffuses back slowly into the bloodstream when the plasma concentration declines. Some absorption can occur from buccal tablets.

Occasionally when an intramuscular injection of progesterone is given, the patient tastes it in her mouth within three minutes. This is due to the rapid metabolism of progesterone, the metabolite pregnanediol being excreted from the lungs (Dalton, 1964).

Progestogens

When progesterone was first isolated it was recognised that it stimulated the endometrium and on withdrawal endometrial bleeding occurred. Biochemists then sought substances which could mimic this action of progesterone and they synthesised progesterone-like compounds called progestogens which caused withdrawal endometrial bleeding when administered to immature oestrogenised rabbits (the Clauberg test). Progestogens are effective when given by mouth or by long-acting injections. Some, such as D-norgesterol, are 2000 times more potent than natural progesterone. Today more is known about the other actions of progesterone and the specificity of steroid transport, and it is recognised that progestogens are not substitutes for natural progesterone.

Fig. 10.4 shows in diagrammatic form the formulae of common

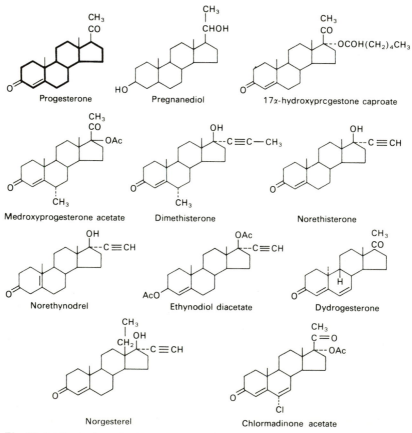

Fig. 10.4 Formulae of progesterone and common progestogens. (From *Principles of Gynaecology* (1975), Jeffcote, Sir N. p 691, Fig 599, London, Butterworth.)

synthetic progestogens, with each steroid molecule containing three benzene rings of six carbon atoms. In three dimensions, however, these formulae may appear as completely different shapes. To illustrate this one only has to consider the benzene rings which can take on the shape of a boat (Fig. 10.5B) or of a chair (Fig. 10.5C). When a boat is attached to a chair it will have a completely different three-dimensional shape from a boat attached to another boat.

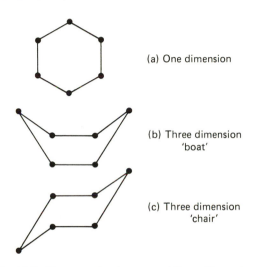

(a) One dimension

(b) Three dimension 'boat'

(c) Three dimension 'chair'

Fig. 10.5   Benzene ring in one and three dimensions.

Furthermore, any extra radicals – for example, OH, CH_3 – added to the benzene ring can be attached above or below the plane of the ring and this again will alter the three-dimensional shape. The three-dimensional structure of progesterone is shown in Fig. 10.6.

A molecule of free progesterone in the intercellular fluid can bind to a progesterone receptor on the cell membrane and the receptor-progesterone complex is transported to the nucleus. The shape of this receptor is specifically matched to bind precisely to the three-dimensional shape of progesterone. A synthetic progestogen may be sufficiently similar in shape to progesterone to latch on to a progesterone receptor in the endometrium and mimic the action of progesterone there, yet be sufficiently different not to bind precisely to progesterone receptors in other

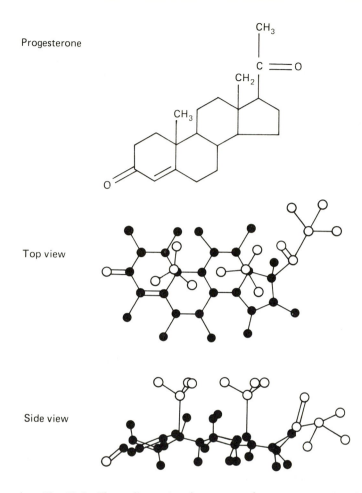

Fig. 10.6   Three-dimensional structure of progesterone.

parts of the body, such as the midbrain. The progestogens may appear similar to other steroids and bind to other binding sites – for instance, norgesterol binds to SHBG, like testosterone and oestradiol.

It must be appreciated that the synthetic long-acting injections of 17-hydroxyprogesterone hexanoate and 17-hydroxyprogesterone caproate are not the same as the naturally occurring 17-hydroxyprogesterone, which is an inactive metabolite of progesterone.

Differences

Whereas progesterone causes secretory changes in the endometrium, the progestogens cause accelerated glandular response leading to secretory exhaustion. This may be a useful property in gynaecological disorders, such as endometriosis and menorrhagia.

Before the advent of the contraceptive pill, norethisterone was known as norethinyl testosterone. Some of the progestogens, particularly the testosterone derivatives and 19 norsteroids (such as ethisterone, dimethisterone, norethynodrel and norethisterone) are androgenic, while others (such as dydrogesterone) are free from androgenic effects. Some progestogens (norethisterone acetate and norethynodrel) have oestrogenic activity which is absent in others (medroxyprogesterone). Progesterone is thermogenic, raising the basal body temperature, while most progestogens do not possess this action, although ethisterone is mildly thermogenic. Progesterone is not anabolic although some progestogens are.

Progesterone causes a reduction in sodium and water retention while progestogens, especially norethisterone, cause an increase in sodium and water retention (Jenkins). Progesterone is synthesised in the adrenal cortex into corticosteroids. Progestogens cannot be synthesised into other corticosteroids in the adrenal cortex.

The major metabolite of progesterone is pregnanediol, but this is not found after the metabolism of progestogens.

One function of progesterone is the maintenance of pregnancy (Rothchild) and when administered after ovulation it assists conception, especially in the cases of defective luteal phase (Jones). The most valuable contribution of the progestogens has been with contraception when administered from the fifth day of the cycle to inhibit ovulation. Most (except dydrogesterone) inhibit ovulation, and also increase the viscosity of the cervical mucus.

When progesterone is administered during pregnancy it has no detrimental effect on the fetus; indeed, surveys have shown that it may result in enhanced intelligence and educational attainment in the child of that pregnancy (Chapter 12) (Dalton). In contrast, when progestogens – particularly the 19 norsteroids and testosterone derivatives – have been administered during early pregnancy it has resulted in masculinisation of the female fetus (Wilkins).

Progesterone is not carcinogenic; in fact, it has been successfully used in the treatment of stilboestrol-associated vaginal adenocarcinoma (Herbert *et al.*). Even so, there is a group of progestogens which are suspected of being carcinogenic because they have produced breast tumours in beagle dogs, a species prone to develop breast tumours. This has resulted in two progestogens, chlormadinone and megestrol, being withdrawn from the market.

Progesterone raises the SHBG binding capacity levels (Dalton M. E.) whereas progestogens decrease the SHBG levels (Granger *et al.*, Victor *et al.*).

Effect of progestogens on the progesterone plasma concentration

Perhaps the most important difference from the therapeutic angle is the fact that the administration of progestogens has been shown to lower the progesterone blood level (Johansson). Fig. 10.7 shows plasma concentrations of progesterone during the luteal phase of a normal cycle compared with concentrations in the same woman during treatment with 30mg medroxyprogesterone acetate daily for 12 days. This effect is dose-dependent, with an even more pronounced lowering of progesterone plasma levels when 60mg were administered.

Similar effects on the reduction of plasma progesterone have been demonstrated following the administration of norethisterone, d-norgesterel and dydrogesterone (Johansson, Kerr). The differences between progesterone and progestogens are given in Table 10.1. Both are valuable in therapeutics but they are not interchangeable, progestogens not being just a convenient synthetic oral substitute for progesterone, and they should have no place in the treatment of premenstrual syndrome or the maintenance of pregnancy.

Many gynaecologists have been concerned by the recent increase in ectopic pregnancies, and it has been suggested but not confirmed that this may be connected with the widespread use of progestogens and the changes it induces in the cervical mucus.

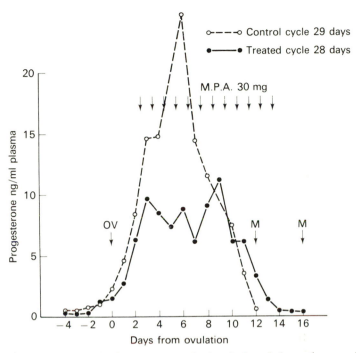

Fig. 10.7 Plasma levels of progesterone during the luteal phase of a normal cycle compared with the levels in the same woman during treatment with 30mg medroxyprogesterone acetate daily for 12 days. (From Johansson E.D.B. (1971). *Amer. J. Obs. Gynecol.* 110; **4**:470.)

Oral contraception

Progestogens are an essential component of the contraceptive pill, either in combination with oestrogen or as the progestogen-only pill. When it is appreciated that progestogen lowers the blood progsterone level, it is readily understood why sufferers from the premenstrual syndrome, who benefit when their progesterone blood level is raised, so often have difficulty in tolerating the pill, which merely serves to increase the severity of their symptoms (Tables 3.3, 27.8 & 27.9).

As a 30-year-old mother wrote, 'I have tried nine types of the pill, but they all make me worse. After a few days I become cross, unhappy, anxious and emotional – at such times I find the baby's

Table 10.1

Differences between progesterone and progestogens

	Progesterone	Progestogen
Occurrence	Naturally occurring	Synthetic
Route of administration	i.m. injections, rectal, vaginal and implantation	Oral and long-acting injections
Clauberg test	Positive, used as standard	Potent, up to ×2000
Effect on endometrium	Change from proliferative to secretory type	Accelerated response followed by secretory exhaustion
Oestrogenic	No	Some
Androgenic	No	Some, especially 19 norsteroids and testosterone derivatives
Anabolic	No	Some
Thermogenic	Yes	Few mildly
Major metabolite	Pregnanediol	Not pregnanediol
Effect on fetus in early pregnancy	Intellectual enhancement	Masculinisation of female
Carcinogenic	None	Some, those carcinogenic in beagle dogs have been withdrawn
SHBG binding capacity	Raised	Lowered

crying unbearable and just throw her into the cot if she won't shut up.'

Another mother of two children wrote, 'Every month for about three days after starting the pill I get symptoms of depression and anxiety, lack of concentration and feel as if my metabolism is being thrown out of gear. I get muzzy heads, my thoughts are out of proportion and I cannot make decisions. Then suddenly I stop the pills and it is as if something clicks into place and I feel well again for a few days.'

Some women on oral contraceptives find that they remove the severe episode of premenstrual tension only to substitute it for a low-grade depression throughout the month, and it is not until they stop the pill for some other reason that they appreciate the general deterioration in their moods which occurred while on oral contraceptives. It is for this reason that many husbands have dissuaded their wives from taking the pill.

11

Treatment of moderate premenstrual syndrome

Premenstrual syndrome is 'the recurrence of symptoms in the premenstruum with absence of symptoms in the postmenstruum'.

Premenstrual syndrome has an individual but specific presentation in each woman and treatment needs careful and personal consideration because of the variety of symptoms and their severity, the variations in cycle length and duration of menstruation, the age, parity, occupation and domestic circumstances – all these need evaluating.

Not all women with premenstrual syndrome require treatment; mild premenstrual symptoms may be a valuable warning of approaching menstruation. A local councillor, for example, who was totally blind, complained bitterly when energetic treatment had completely removed her premenstrual symptoms and she started unexpectedly to menstruate at a public function.

Women deserving of treatment for premenstrual syndrome are those whose symptoms are causing unnecessary suffering and interfering with their normal lifestyle, domestic or marital life.

Progesterone is the treatment for those with severe premenstrual syndrome, but non-hormonal treatment should be given to women whose symptoms are mild or moderately severe and to those who are completing a menstrual chart to confirm the diagnosis; it should also be given to women with menstrual distress and only minor exacerbations of premenstrual syndrome. Fig. 11.1 shows the scheme for treatment in those with diagnosed premenstrual syndrome.

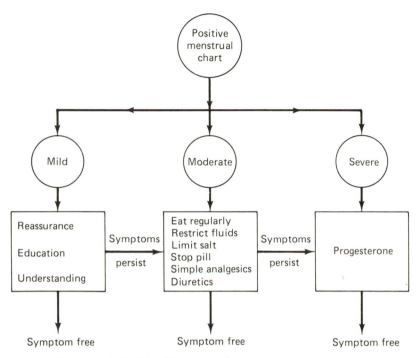

Fig. 11.1   Schedule of treatment for premenstrual syndrome.

Reassurance of menstrual chart

Encouraging the patient to record the dates of symptoms and menstruation for a few months is always worth while. This reassures the patient, as she sees for herself that although the chronic symptoms recur there is always a phase free from symptoms in each cycle. Too often her visit to the doctor is accompanied by a hidden fear that the joint pains are an early sign of crippling arthritis, or that the headaches doom her to a painful death from a cerebral tumour. A chart may be particularly useful for the woman with recurrent upper respiratory infection who is demanding monthly supplies of antibiotics. Once the allergic and non-infectious nature of her rhinitis is appreciated she may be able to accept a prophylactic course of mild antihistamine drugs.

Self-help treatment

Once the patient recognises that she has mild premenstrual syndrome she should be taught to adjust her lifestyle to the cyclical problem. It should be explained to her that during the premenstruum she should avoid heavy supermarket trips and exhausting outings. Instead, she should enjoy social and dinner engagements, TV and hi-fi. The woman will also need reassuring that after menstruation she will have all the energy she needs to do the work that she has left undone during the premenstruum. She should also aim at having extra rest with earlier bedtimes and spells of relaxation during the day. Today many young mothers have learnt the art of relaxation for childbirth and can use these exercises at home. She may prefer to do this alone at home or to join one of the 'Relaxation for Living' classes locally; yoga is also beneficial.

Avoidance of long intervals between food

In Chapter 5 the effect of relative hypoglycaemia was discussed. The sudden changes of mood, panic attacks, aggressive outbursts, migraine and epilepsy all tend to occur when there has been a long gap between taking carbohydrates, usually exceeding five hours in the day or 13 hours overnight. It is therefore worth advising patients to eat little and often, aiming at some carbohydrate intake every three hours during the daytime and ten hours overnight. This means dividing the usual three daily meals into six snacks – it does not mean increasing the total daily intake of food. Patients should be advised to have a smaller breakfast, but add biscuits or a sandwich at elevenses, a smaller lunch but add a cake at teatime, and leave the dessert from supper to have at bedtime. Even those on a weight-reducing diet of 900 calories can easily divide it into six snacks of 150 calories each. The popular high-fibre diet lends itself easily to the division into six snacks daily. It is better to alter the diet throughout the month rather than only in the premenstruum.

Restriction of fluid and salt

The restriction of fluid intake to one pint daily has advantages for those with marked water retention. It is surprising how many women spend all day drinking tea or coffee during the premenstruum mistakenly hoping it will give them a little more energy. Many people do not appreciate the high content of salt and monosodium gluconate in convenience foods and savoury snacks. Advice is needed on the limitation of high salt-containing foods and the avoidance of salt supplementation at the table.

Correction of constipation

Constipation is an almost universal accompaniment of the premenstrual syndrome and simple correction is beneficial. Modern diets are low in roughage and many people can benefit from the addition of two tablespoons of bran to their daily diet, and also from increasing their consumption of fresh fruit and vegetables. In India there is a custom for all women to take a dose of magnesium sulphate during the premenstruum to relieve the body of accumulated poisons. It is fascinating to find how often ancient customs turn out to be of value, although not always in the way that the ancients envisaged. There is much to commend their use of magnesium sulphate as both a laxative and a dehydrating agent.

Stop oral contraception

All oral contraceptives contain progestogens, some also contain oestrogen. As was emphasised in Chapter 10, the oral synthetic progestogens lower blood progesterone level so causing a deterioration in premenstrual syndrome. The oestrogen-containing pills cause a further deterioration of the oestrogen-progesterone ratio, thus again increasing the severity of premenstrual syndrome. Hence all types of oral contraception should be stopped (Fig. 11.2). The question of the most suitable method of contraception needs to be considered individually for some other method is needed. Bilateral tubal litigation is not advised because this too has been shown to result in lowering the blood progesterone level (Radwanska *et al.*). (Fig. 3.16).

Psychotherapy

Clare (1982) reminds us that there has been no study to date of the therapeutic efficacy of altering women's attitudes to pre-

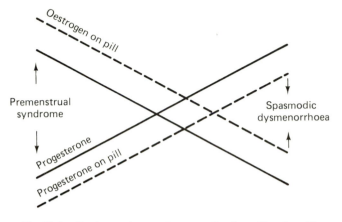

Fig. 11.2   Oestrogen/progesterone ratio altered by the pill.

menstrual syndrome and menstrual experiences. The efficacy of psychotherapy remains doubtful in the treatment of pre-menstrual syndrome and there is no evidence that patients with severe premenstrual syndrome benefit from acupuncture. At the Sixth International Congress of Psychosomatic Obstetrics and Gynaecology, held in Berlin in September 1980, the overall conclusion was that premenstrual syndrome must be regarded as an endocrinopathy (van Keep & Utian).

Drug therapy

The previous drug therapy given to 256 new patients with severe premenstrual syndrome seen in 1981 and 1982 is shown in Table 11.1. Tranquillisers (63%) and anti-depressant drugs (53%) failed to ease the symptoms of these patients. The 25 women (9%) who had previously received progesterone were referred either because of incorrect dosage or diagnosis, or for reassurance for the referring doctor that progesterone therapy was the correct approach (see also Appendix Table 27.12).

While keeping a menstrual chart to confirm the diagnosis and to determine the precise days on which the symptoms are present all progestogens, oestrogens and oral contraceptives should be stopped. Most of the other medications can be limited to the premenstruum, except for the antidepressants which need to be taken throughout the cycle because several

Table 11.1

Previous medication for premenstrual syndrome

	236 patients first seen in 1981 and 1982	
	n	%
Tranquillisers	173	63
Antidepressants	146	53
Progestogens	75	27
Pyridoxine	58	21
Diuretics	58	21
Oral contraceptives	32	12
Analgesics	31	11
Progesterone	25	9
Oestrogens	22	8
Hormone preparations	22	8
Prostaglandin inhibitors	10	4
Bromocriptine	8	3

days elapse before their full effect is felt. While patients are following dietary and other instructions for the relief of premenstrual syndrome their other drug medication can be gradually reduced and finally stopped. Each drug reduction should occur in the postmenstruum and never during the premenstruum.

Diuretics

Diuretics are a simple method of helping the patient with mild premenstrual symptoms that are due to water retention, but they will not help the psychological symptoms, and indeed they may increase the lethargy. The choice, therefore, should be one of the slower acting potassium-sparing diuretics, preferably used on alternate days from ovulation to menstruation. If only partial benefit is obtained, there is a natural temptation to increase the dosage and frequency, and to change to the quick-acting diuretics. The course then gets extended and electrolyte imbalance occurs. By this time the patient is often addicted to diuretics and claims that she gets bloated if they are stopped for only one day. As one patient explained, 'But I can even hear the water splashing about in my stomach'.

Potassium

Potassium depletion may be suspected in those giving a history of prolonged diuretic administration, food cravings, prolonged dieting, and those complaining of lethargy and muscle weakness throughout the cycle.

Potassium, either as effervescent or enteric-coated tablets, should be given sufficient to maintain the potassium level above the lower level of normal to an optimum level of 4.0 to 4.3mmol/1.

Spironolactone

It was hoped that spironolactone, an aldosterone antagonist, would prove helpful in this syndrome (O'Brien *et al.*), but these hopes have not been fulfilled in practice (Smith). If used, it is best given as a combination tablet with a diuretic, and although it is claimed to be potassium-sparing it is advisable to have regular potassium estimations done and give a potassium supplement if indicated.

Antidepressants

Antidepressants would appear to be the first line of treatment for the premenstrual depression, but in practice it is among this group of women that most of the failures are noticed, possibly because tricyclic antidepressants raise the prolactin level and thus lower the progesterone blood level. Doses of tricyclics, which are effective in other patients, tend to increase the premenstrual lethargy and therefore make them unacceptable. The tricyclic group of drugs take about two weeks to have their full effect, which means that if they are used they should be given during the symptom-free two weeks in the hope of helping the two depressed weeks. For premenstrual depressives, lithium is sometimes claimed to be a useful drug for easing mood swings and depression, and may be used simultaneously with progesterone therapy if needed. The most useful antidepressives are the monoamine oxidase inhibitors (MAOI), but they do require dietary restrictions. Their action is quite rapid and so they can be limited to the premenstruum.

Progestogens

Chapter 10 dealt with the differences between progesterone and progestogens, and explained how most of the actions required of progesterone in the treatment of premenstrual syndrome were not present in progestogens. Progestogens should NOT be regarded as routine treatment for premenstrual syndrome; however, there are a few conditions in which they can be used beneficially.

Patients with presenting symptoms of engorged and tender breasts premenstrually often benefit from the androgenic progestogens, such as norethisterone, in doses of 5–15mg daily from ovulation to the onset of menstruation. If necessary, diuretics may be given simultaneously. Posthysterectomy patients with cyclical lower abdominal pains, and possibly a history of endometriosis, may benefit from continuous norethisterone 10–30mg daily in courses of six months with a gradual reduction over the year (p. 227).

Pyridoxine

In 1974 Giles in Australia found many patients attending his clinic with functional gynaecological disorders, who had mistakenly been found to have low plasma pyridoxine concentrations. This suggested that low pyridoxine might give rise to premenstrual syndrome, so pyridoxine was prescribed. When it was later found that the assays were faulty, his clinic stopped prescribing pyridoxine. Nevertheless, elsewhere throughout the world it is still being prescribed.

Pyridoxine (Vitamin B6) deficiency causes lethargy, depression and irritability, but this deficiency is not limited to the premenstruum, if there is any vitamin deficiency it will persist throughout the month. Pyridoxine is valuable for those who have developed a deficiency of pyridoxine while on oestrogen-containing contraceptives or after oestrogen therapy at the menopause.

Pyridoxine is a cheap and harmless remedy and may usefully be prescribed as a therapeutic trial while a patient is recording her symptoms to confirm the diagnosis of premenstrual syndrome. If a patient does benefit from pyridoxine, it is the physician's responsibility to investigate her diet carefully to ensure that she is not suffering from other vitamin deficiencies. Mineral, vitamin and essential fatty acid supplements are often recommended (Abraham, Horrobin, Brush) but they are of no use for premenstrual syndrome. Any such deficiencies will be present throughout the cycle and may cause menstrual distress but not premenstrual syndrome.

Bromocriptine

Bromocriptine has been advocated for the treatment of premenstrual syndrome (Benedek-Jaszmann & Hearn-Sturtevant). Its place in lowering prolactin levels is undisputed and it has proved effective in amenorrhoea-galactorrhoea syndrome and in the inhibition of lactation. In premenstrual syndrome it has been most successful where there is breast engorgement and generalised oedema and for women with a recent history of puerperal depression, in whom it may bring relief regardless of whether or not the prolactin levels are raised (Graham *et al.*). The side effects include nausea and vomiting (particularly if taken without food), headaches, insomnia, confusion and an increase in libido. The usual dose is 2.5mg bromocriptine at night with food from day 10 until the onset of menstruation. This dose can then gradually be increased by monthly increments up to 7.5mg. In patients already on progesterone therapy it may be started gradually, initially with progesterone, and then the progesterone should gradually be reduced while increasing the bromocriptine.

Recent double-blind controlled trials in 13 patients using 2.5mg bromocriptine or identical placebo tablets failed to show any significant difference in the alleviation of premenstrual mood swings, swelling or headaches (Ghose & Coppen).

12

Principles of progesterone therapy

It must first be appreciated that progesterone treatment is essentially *prophylactic*. If it is administered too late other reactions will have occurred which cannot be corrected by progesterone (Fig. 12.1).

Thus progesterone prophylactic treatment is indicated in the following conditions:

1. *Premenstrual syndrome,* from ovulation until menstruation – that is, before symptoms have developed (Chapter 13).
2. *Defective luteal phase* in infertility, starting treatment after ovulation but before progesterone would have reached the mid-luteal peak (Chapter 22).
3. *Habitual abortion,* starting from confirmation of pregnancy and continuing until full placental production has occurred (Chapter 22).
4. *Threatened abortion,* starting when hyperemesis or pregnancy symptoms occur (Chapter 22).
5. *Pre-eclampsia,* starting during the symptomatic stage and before the development of oedema, weight gain or proteinuria (Chapter 20).
6. *Postnatal depression,* starting immediately after the completion of labour and continuing until the first menstruation (Chapter 21).

Progesterone treatment is also valuable in the following:

1. Cyclical symptoms at the menopause and in patients after hysterectomy (Chapter 23).
2. Stilboestrol-associated vaginal adenosis (Herbert *et al.*).

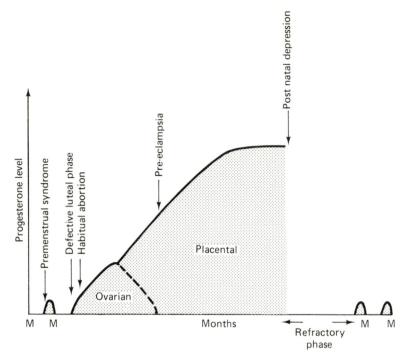

Fig. 12.1   Times of starting prophylactic progesterone treatment.

Safety and efficacy

In 1983 a public inquiry was held by the Federal Drug Administration in Washington into progesterone therapy in premenstrual syndrome. To provide the necessary information on the safety and efficacy of progesterone two research assistants extracted details from the files of all patients seen by the author, in 1982 who had received progesterone. Due to shortage of time the evidence submitted covered information only on those women whose surnames began with A–H or W–Z; further particulars are contained in the Appendix. Of the 1006 files scrutinised 610 (61%) had received progesterone and information about these patients is contained in this and other chapters of the book (Dalton, 1983).

Methods of progesterone administration

1. Intramuscular injection (Chapter 15).
2. Rectal suppository (Chapter 14).

3. Vaginal pessary (Chapter 14).
4. Implantation (Chapter 16).
5. Local application.
6. Buccal sublingual tablets.

Oral progesterone is not very effective because progesterone receptors in the liver metabolise the progesterone before it reaches the systemic circulation.

The preferred method of administration in 565 women with severe premenstrual syndrome seen in 1982 was, suppositories or pessaries in 490 (87%), intramuscular injections in 50 (9%) and 25 (4%) received an implant (Table 12.1) (see also Table 27.13).

Table 12.1

Method of progesterone administration

	n=565	
	n	%
Suppositories	490	87
Injections	50	9
Implant	25	4

Rectal injections of a progesterone solution have been tried; they have no advantage over the rectal suppositories other than being cheaper to produce. Larger and more frequent doses of the solution may be required. To date there are no absorption studies of progesterone rectal solution.

Local progesterone

There are only a few instances where local progesterone may be used with good effect; in most cases the patients are polysymptomatic and systemic treatment by transdermal application requires very high dosage of progesterone. Nasal drops (10%) may be used in the treatment of premenstrual rhinitis, and progesterone cream (10%) may be used for premenstrual vaginal and vulval ulceration. In all cases the local pharmacist will need to supply the preparation. Progesterone gel is available in France, where it is recommended for premenstrual mastitis if there are no other systemic symptoms.

Buccal administration

Sublingual tablets of progesterone can be absorbed systemically and do cause a rise in blood progesterone level. While they are being used, however, the woman is instructed not to swallow, eat or talk, so using them three times daily has been found to be an impossible task for all except contemplative nuns.

Dosage

Dosages of 25–100mg daily may be used intramuscularly, while the suppositories and pessaries are available in doses of 200 and 400mg and may be used up to four times daily as their absorption is more rapid (Fig. 13.2) (Nillius & Johansson). It is rarely necessary to increase the injections above 100mg daily in the non-pregnant woman, although it may be raised to 300mg daily during pregnancy or in the immediate postpartum.

When pellets of pure progesterone are implanted, 5–16 pellets of 100mg may be used.

When patients are already taking progesterone they may take an extra emergency dose should they feel that an attack is imminent. An injection of 50–100mg will usually give a boost within 30–60 minutes and the benefit from a 400mg suppository or pessary will often be appreciated within 20–30 minutes.

The dosage required tends to be higher among parous women, those of slim build and those with a history of pre-eclampsia. This does not appear to be related to age, severity or multiplicity of symptoms. After a pregnancy it will be necessary to re-establish the dose required. Women who have had a good pregnancy and puerperium may not need progesterone therapy again.

Continuous progesterone therapy

The reasons for continuous progesterone therapy in 78 of the 610 women (13%) seen in 1982 is shown in Table 12.2. Hysterectomy and/or oophorectomy accounted for the largest group of 38 women (49%), and menopause for 16 women (20%). The 11 women (14%) with premenstrual syndrome receiving continuous progesterone treatment were on that regimen either because they were postponing menstruation for a specific event, such as competitions, examinations or trips abroad, or because progesterone (and often an earlier implant) had produced amenorrhoea and they were then frightened that the symptoms would reappear with the return of menstruation. In these latter cases the dose of progesterone should be gradually reduced until menstruation is re-established.

Continuous progesterone therapy was also used in the puerperium until the return of menstruation. The regimen of progesterone in postnatal depression is discussed in Chapter 21.

Table 12.2

Reasons for continuous progesterone therapy (suppositories or injections)

Reason	n=78 n	%
PMS	11	14
Pregnant	3	4
PND	4	5
Prophylactic PND	6	8
Menopause	16	20
Hysterectomy/oophorectomy	38	49

Overdose

The progesterone level in pregnancy rises some 20–30 times higher than the peak level during the luteal phase (Johansson). In pregnancy this raised level of progesterone is maintained – not just for two weeks as in a menstrual cycle, but continuously for a full nine months (Figure 12.1). It is therefore impossible to overdose a parous woman with progesterone, because she will already have experienced considerably higher levels of progesterone in pregnancy than it is possible to administer either by injections or suppositories. Most nulliparous women are quite capable of withstanding the high levels of progesterone, such as are expected in pregnancy. It is only the very immature woman who might notice the effects of overdosage, which are euphoria, restless energy, faintness and uterine cramps.

Progesterone suppositories and pessaries may be given to women who are known to have attempted an overdose because they cannot overdose with them. Only one suppository or pessary can be inserted into an orifice at a time – or within one hour – because otherwise the wax will prevent further absorption. A rectal and a vaginal suppository may be used simultaneously.

Side effects

There are no serious side effects. There may be alterations in the length of the cycle. If the cycle is lengthened then the progesterone should be stopped at the time of the expected onset and menstruation may be expected within 48 hours. Occasionally there is a shortening of the cycle, which can be corrected by starting future courses of progesterone a day or two later.

Premenstrual spotting may occur, especially if progesterone is started during the follicular phase. This is best dealt with by stopping progesterone to allow menstruation to occur and then starting the next course a day or two later, not in the follicular phase.

If a course of progesterone has been started and then inadvertently stopped, menstruation may be expected to begin within 48 hours. This may happen when the patient has an unexpected weekend away from home, or if the nurse fails to give the injection on Sundays. Thus erratic progesterone takers have erratic menstruations.

Some women develop amenorrhoea with progesterone, especially when it is continued for many months. As they are by this time symptom free, however, many women prefer to remain on a continuous but gradually reducing dose of progesterone. Amenorrhoea may continue for a long time, in some cases as long as five years.

A generalised urticarial rash may occur as a reaction to the oily solution of progesterone injections. Treatment should continue with suppositories or pessaries.

Women who are below the average weight for their height and age may find they gain weight on progesterone, while those who are overweight for their height and age often lose weight on progesterone.

Perhaps it needs to be emphasised that, unlike the synthetic progestogens, the natural progesterone does not cause any rise in blood pressure; indeed, in sufferers from premenstrual syndrome who develop a rise premenstrually it may reduce the blood pressure (see Figs. 7.10 and 7.12) (Dalton, 1954). In addition, progesterone does not interfere with the blood clotting mechanisms such as occurs with oestrogen administration.

Progesterone has no carcinogenic effects, and indeed is used in the treatment of some forms – for example, corrections of vaginal adenosis after stilboestrol (DES) administration in fetal life (Herbert *et al.*).

No cases of addiction to progesterone have been encountered, although a few women do use up to 8×400mg suppositories daily. These tend to be women with very low SHBG levels, which show only a slow rise during progesterone administration and barely reach normal levels. This suggests that the absorption of progesterone is poor, rather than that there is any abuse of medication. Generally, if there is poor absorption with suppositories then injections are used, but some women find it inconvenient to visit the doctor daily or have the nurse call daily at an unspecified time and prefer to be in charge of their own medication, even if it means using suppositories frequently each day.

Long-term effects
The duration of progesterone therapy is given in Table 12.3. No adverse effects have been noted during the constant monitoring of 120 women who have had continuous progesterone therapy for five years, nor in 19 women who have been on progesterone therapy for over 15 years (see also Appendix Tables 27.15, 27.16, 27.28 & 27.29).

A raised glucose tolerance curve was found in a few women, particularly among those with amenorrhoea following an implant or after a hysterectomy, but there have been no new cases of diabetes in these, or in any progesterone-treated women, during the past 30 years. One woman developed diabetes 8 years after stopping progesterone treatment (Table 27.17). The 28-year-old mother with premenstrual epilepsy, whose chart is shown in Fig. 5.3, had an oral glucose tolerance test (dose 1gm/kg=72.6gm) before starting progesterone treatment. These tests were repeated over the following two years and the last one showed mildly abnormal glucose levels (Fig. 12.2).

Long-term effect of antenatal progesterone
A 20-year survey of children whose mothers received antenatal progesterone given before the 16th week showed that they had increased intelligence (Dalton, 1968 & 1976).

Attention was focused on this possibility by a chance remark: 'How curious that so many of your patients are among the brightest at the local school.' Looking at the antenatal records of the mothers of these children it was noted that all had received progesterone for pregnancy symptoms during that pregnancy. A simple pilot study was arranged by the local medical officer and

Table 12.3

Date of commencement of progesterone therapy

	n=610		
1–5 years	1982	133	
	1981	143	
	1980	96	
	1979	76	
	1978	51	n=490
6–10 years	1977	25	
	1976	13	
	1975	14	
	1974	10	
	1973	11	n=73
11–15 years	1972	12	
	1971	6	
	1970	6	
	1969	4	
	1968	0	n=28
16–20 years	1967	3	
	1966	2	
	1965	2	
	1964	2	
	1963	1	n=10
21–35 years	1960	3	
	1959	2	
	1956	1	
	1953	1	
	1952	1	
	1948	1	n=9

the results were encouraging. Later examination, by community physicians and health visitors, at the first birthday of both progesterone children and controls born at the Chase Farm Hospital during the controlled trials into the prophylactic value of progesterone in the treatment of pre-eclampsia, provided further evidence of earlier standing and walking among the children whose mothers had taken progesterone (Fig. 12.3).

A follow-up at the City of London Maternity Hospital was then organised using the labour ward register, in which each

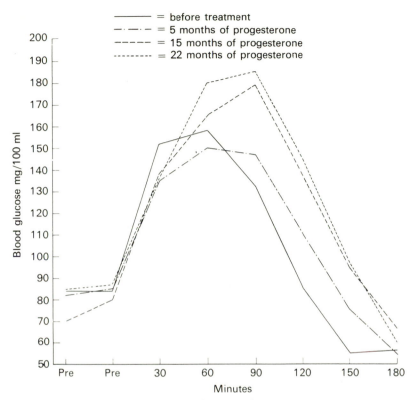

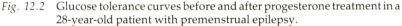

Fig. 12.2   Glucose tolerance curves before and after progesterone treatment in a 28-year-old patient with premenstrual epilepsy.

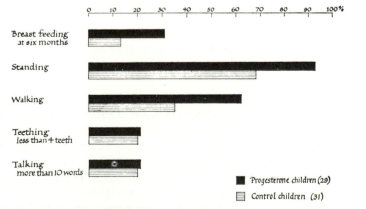

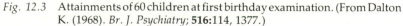

Fig. 12.3   Attainments of 60 children at first birthday examination. (From Dalton K. (1968). *Br. J. Psychiatry;* **516:**114, 1377.)

progesterone child was matched with the next-born normal control child and with a child whose mother had developed pre-eclampsia. The respective head teachers were asked to assess the named child's ability as 'average', 'above' or 'below' in English, verbal reasoning, arithmetic, craft work and physical education (Fig. 12.4).

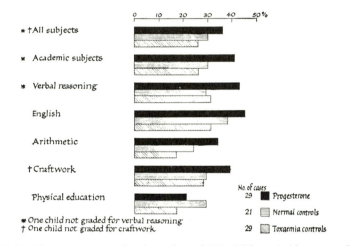

Fig. 12.4 Above-average school grades of 79 children 9–10 years. (From Dalton K. (1968). *Br. J. Psychiatry*; **516:** 114, 1377.)

The results showed that more progesterone children than controls were regarded as above average in the academic subjects, English, verbal reasoning and arithmetic.

Furthermore, among the progesterone children the results were dose-dependent, being best among those in whom administration began before the 16th week (Fig. 12.5), and with a dose exceeding 8g (Fig. 12.6).

A follow-up of these children, when aged 18 to 20 years, showed that the progesterone children stayed at school longer, obtaining more 'O' levels and 'A' levels and 11 (32%) of the 34 progesterone children obtained university places compared with 6% of controls, 6% of children in the Borough of Haringey, where most of the children lived, and 6% for the Inner London Education Authority. Again, the effect of the progesterone was dose-dependent, being best when administered before the 16th week in high doses for longer than 8 weeks (Fig. 12.7 and 12.8).

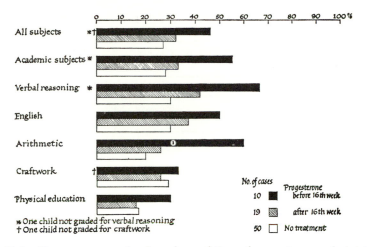

Fig. 12.5 Above-average school grades and time of progesterone administration. (From Dalton K. (1968). *Br. J. Psychiatry*; **516**:114, 1377).

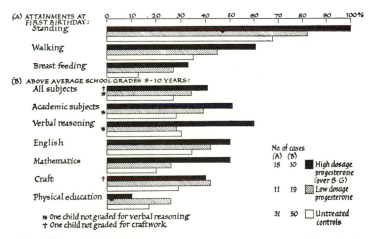

Fig. 12.6 Effect of high-dosage progesterone on attainments. (From Dalton K. (1968). *Br. J. Psychiatry*; **516**:114, 1377.)

Zussman and Zussman, psychologists from Stanford University, gave a full two-hour testing to 30 of these progesterone children and concluded that there was a clear advantage in the differential aptitude test in numerical ability and marginally significant relationship with spatial and mechanical ability in relation to the dose of progesterone received. The Bem sex-role

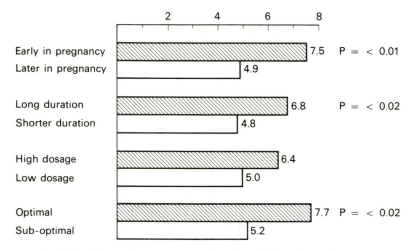

Fig. 12.7   Effect of progesterone dosage on 'O' level examinations.

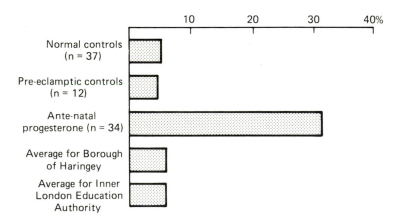

Fig. 12.8   University entrance gained by progesterone children and controls.

inventory and the Californian Psychological Inventory did not relate significantly with masculinity or femininity score.

Lynch and colleagues from Keele University expressed interest in the findings and were given every assistance to enable them to follow-up the progesterone and control children whose mothers were included in the two controlled trials into the use of progesterone in the prophylaxis of pre-eclampsia. The children of the mothers who received progesterone by injection were then 16

years of age, and the children whose mothers received progesterone by suppository were two years of age. In these trials no
progesterone was administered before the 16th week, and
women with pregnancy symptoms between the 16th and 28th
week of pregnancy were allocated at random to the progesterone
or control groups. Less than 20% of the children were traced, but
they found no differences between the progesterone and control
groups in their mental or social development, or their spatial,
perceptual or personality tests. As none of these mothers received
progesterone before the 16th week, this suggests that the
beneficial effect of progesterone is limited to those receiving
early administration of progesterone. So, as with rubella and
thalidamide, there may be a period of maximal sensitivity to
progesterone during the first 16 weeks when the fetal brain is
developing, but in this case the effect is beneficial and is clear
evidence that there are no long-term side effects from progesterone administered in pregnancy.

Contraindications

There are no absolute contraindications to progesterone therapy.
Nevertheless, if candidiasis is present progesterone may cause an
exacerbation of the infection; thus if there is a past history of
vaginal infection or if there is a vaginal discharge it is a wise
precaution to give a course of antifungal agent before starting, or
simultaneously with, the initial course of progesterone.

It is best to avoid rectal suppositories if there is a history of faecal
incontinence or colitis.

It should also be emphasised that there are no contraindications
to the use of progesterone during a pregnancy or the puerperium.
No fetal abnormalities result from its use in pregnancy.

Drug interactions

No drug interactions have been noticed with progesterone. When
progesterone is first given it is as well to leave the patient on any
medications which she is already receiving, such as steroids,
anti-convulsants, anti-depressants, bronchodilators or diuretics,
and then gradually reduce the other medication at the end of each
course, eliminating the drug during the postmenstruum if it is
being taken continuously. Progesterone can also be given simultaneously with progestogens, as in patients with endometriosis
receiving nor-ethisterone or danazol.

Legal requirement in the United States

It should be noted that in the United States progesterone and progestogens have not yet been differentiated by the Food and Drug Administration legislation and manufacturers are still required to enclose a 'Patient Package Insert' when dispensing progesterone. Physicians are still required to comply with Federal regulations when prescribing progesterone and give a 'Patient Package Insert' to each premenopausal woman, except those in whom childbearing is impossible. It is hoped these regulations will be altered in the near future.

13

Progesterone therapy for premenstrual syndrome

Premenstrual syndrome is 'the recurrence of symptoms in the pre-menstruum with absence of symptoms in the postmenstruum'.

It is important to appreciate that not all patients with premenstrual syndrome require progesterone therapy, nor is there any justification for treating with hormones those whose symptoms do not warrant such treatment. There are, however, many women whose symptoms can be relieved only with progesterone and these women certainly need treating for their lives can be transformed.

Indications for progesterone treatment in premenstrual syndrome

1. Recurrent symptoms interfering with normal working capacity and lifestyle.
2. Risk of premenstrual assault, suicide, self-injury or alcoholic bout.
3. Marital disharmony and domestic stress resulting from the symptoms.
4. Costly hospital admission is the only alternative.
5. Recurrent conflict with the law threatening a prison sentence.

Menstrual record
It has already been emphasised that the diagnosis of premenstrual syndrome depends on the time relationship of symptoms to

menstruation and not on symptoms alone. It is essential before beginning treatment, therefore, to have an accurate menstrual record and to continue to use it throughout treatment in order to monitor progress. It is a great temptation to start treatment on the evidence of a patient's verbal statement, especially if the symptoms are serious or urgent. Many patients have stated at first interviews that their symptoms are premenstrual and their menstruation is regular with a 28-day cycle and a three-day menstrual loss, only to find, after careful charting the following month, that their symptoms extend until the second day of menstruation in a cycle of 32 days with five days' menstrual loss. Timing is critical and it is attention to these minor alterations in symptoms and cycles that determines the ideal course of treatment for each individual.

The first question to be answered is whether daily supervision is necessary: the answer is always 'yes' in cases where there is even a slight risk of suicide, assault or alcoholic bouts (Fig. 13.1). In such cases daily supervision by a nurse is essential and the patient should receive progesterone by injection.

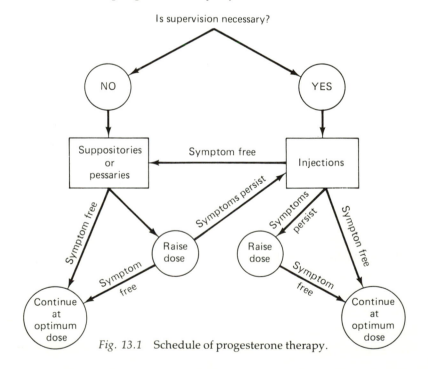

Fig. 13.1   Schedule of progesterone therapy.

With patients in hospital it is usually more convenient to begin treatment with injections, and there will always be those patients who, aesthetically, prefer injections to suppositories or pessaries. In other cases it is usual to start with suppositories or pessaries. If there is no response to the initial dose it is raised, but about 5–10% of patients do not get adequate absorption even from high doses of suppositories or pessaries and in these cases it is necessary to give injections (Tables 12.1, 27.13 & 27.27).

Initial course

The normal course of progesterone therapy is from ovulation to menstruation. Menstrual cycles, however, are very individual and vary from woman to woman and, within limits, from cycle to cycle. This is the reason for emphasising the importance of accurate recording on a menstrual chart, thus enabling each individual to have a personally adjusted course depending on the length of cycle and duration of symptoms.

Progesterone has a cumulative action over the first five days of administration (Nillius & Johansson). In those with symptoms lasting less than seven days, therefore the course of treatment should start five days before the symptoms are expected to occur. If symptoms start at ovulation it is only necessary to start the course two days earlier and continue the treatment until menstruation begins.

If severe symptoms persist during menstruation, treatment may be continued until the full menstrual flow at a lower dose, but by giving a routine premenstrual course of progesterone the menstrual symptoms often do not develop (Fig. 13.2).

Patients who have an unduly long cycle of 35–40 days with symptoms only on the last few days should be given progesterone from day 21 to 28. This will produce menstruation within 24–48 hours of stopping progesterone and therefore before the symptoms might be expected (Fig. 13.3).

The level of SHBG in premenstrual syndrome is dose-related in its response to progesterone (Fig. 13.4) (Dalton M. E.). Thus, if an SHBG estimation is available before starting treatment, it will give an indication whether an individual patient requires a high or low dose.

Starting day of progesterone

The starting day for 535 women with severe premenstrual

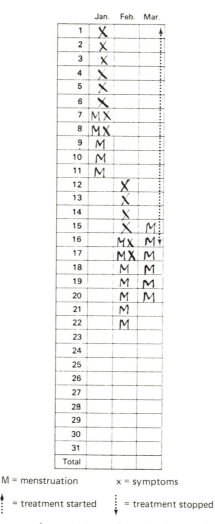

	Jan.	Feb.	Mar.
1	X		▲
2	X		
3	X		
4	X		
5	X		
6	X		
7	M X		
8	M X		
9	M		
10	M		
11	M		
12		X	
13		X	
14		X	
15		X	M
16		M X	M ▼
17		M X	M
18		M	M
19		M	M
20		M	M
21		M	
22		M	
23			
24			
25			
26			
27			
28			
29			
30			
31			
Total			

M = menstruation   x = symptoms

↑ = treatment started   ⋮ = treatment stopped

Fig. 13.2   Initial course of progesterone from day 14 continued until day 2 as symptoms persisted until day 2.

syndrome seen in 1982 is shown in Table 13.1. Those women starting on day 8 are using progesterone contraceptively in a low dose until ovulation, when they will increase to the full dose required for symptomatic relief. Women starting progesterone on days 10–18 are using it from ovulation until menstruation, the earlier ones having short cycles of 21 days. Those women starting on days 18–22 are either anxious to conceive and so start after

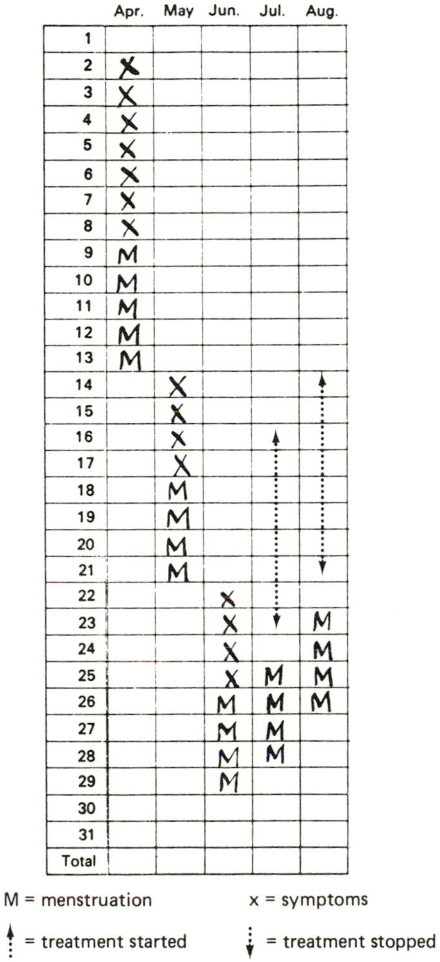

	Apr.	May	Jun.	Jul.	Aug.
1					
2	X				
3	X				
4	X				
5	X				
6	X				
7	X				
8	X				
9	M				
10	M				
11	M				
12	M				
13	M				
14		X			↑
15		X			⋮
16		X		↑	⋮
17		X		⋮	⋮
18		M		⋮	⋮
19		M		⋮	⋮
20		M		⋮	⋮
21		M		⋮	↓
22			X	⋮	
23			X	↓	M
24			X		M
25			X	M	M
26			M	M	M
27			M	M	
28			M	M	
29			M		
30					
31					
Total					

M = menstruation   x = symptoms

↑ = treatment started   ↓ = treatment stopped

Fig. 13.3 Long cycle of 39–40 days with symptoms on days 34–40, treated with progesterone from days 21–28 to shorten the cycle to 30 days and to eliminate symptoms.

ovulation, or women with a short duration of symptoms. The few women starting on day 24 represent either those with short duration of symptoms or those with long cycles who use progesterone for only four days in anticipation of menstruation starting within 48 hours of stopping progesterone (which usually occurs), so shortening the cycle and eliminating the development of symptoms.

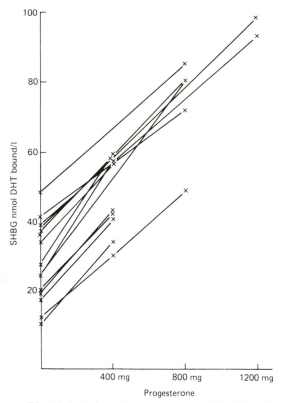

Fig. 13.4   Effect of progesterone on SHBG levels.

Adjustments to the course

After initial treatment, adjustments may need to be made. Those who are symptom-free may have the dose reduced to 200mg suppositories or pessaries. The course may also be progressively reduced in gradations of two days from the initial course of 14 days to the shortest course which brings full symptomatic relief (Fig. 13.5).

Patients who receive partial benefit, noticing relief of symptoms during part of the day only, should be changed to twice daily administration of suppositories or pessaries. Others may have had relief of symptoms during the premenstruum, but with a postponement of symptoms during menstruation, these should be given their normal dose during the premenstruum and half the dose during the first four days of menstruation. Patients who

Table 13.1

Day of starting progesterone

Day	n=540	%
8	36	7
10	9	2
12	37	7
14	299	55
16	36	7
18	19	3
20	9	2
22	7	1
24	5	1
When necessary	5	1
Continuous	78	14

receive no benefit from 400mg suppositories or pessaries should have twice daily administration during the second month, and this may be increased to three or four daily in subsequent months. If there is still no benefit a course of daily injections should be given, 50mg for nulliparous and 100mg for parous patients. If daily injections bring relief, injections may then be given on alternate days, possibly alternating with suppositories on the injection-free day.

After the initial course the patient may be given permission to use an extra suppository or pessary during the day if she feels the need – for example, at times of mounting aggression, panic attacks, impending migraine or unaccountable depression. She should also be advised that if she stops the course prematurely menstruation is likely to follow within 48 hours of the last dose.

It might be mentioned that when treating blind patients, it is better not to aim at complete relief of all symptoms, for they usually prefer some mild symptoms as a warning of the imminence of menstruation; otherwise they may have difficulty in distinguishing a vaginal discharge from menstrual blood which could stain their clothes.

Higher doses are required by women of high parity, a history of pre-eclampsia or postnatal depression and also those of slim build. The dosage of progesterone is not related to age, severity or multiplicity of symptoms.

Restabilisation of the dose is necessary after a pregnancy. If

	Jan.	Feb.	Mar.	Apr.	May	Jun.	Jul.	Aug.	Sep.	Oct.	Nov.	Dec.
1						↑	↑					
2								↑				
3												
4												
5								X				
6								X	↓			
7								X	M			
8								X	M			
9								X↓	M			
10							↓	M	M			
11						M		M				
12				X		↓	M	M				
13			X	X		M	M	M				
14			X	X	↓	M	M					
15			X	X	M	M						
16		X	X	X	M	M						
17		X	X	M	M							
18		X	X	M	M							
19		X	M	M								
20		X	M	M								
21		M	M									
22		M	M									
23		M										
24		M										
25												
26												
27								↑				
28												
29												
30				↑								
31												
Total												

M = menstruation　　　　　　　　　　x = symptoms

↑ = treatment started　　　　　　　↓ = treatment stopped

The initial course of progesterone from Day 14 until the onset of menstruation eliminated symptoms. Subsequent courses of 12 and 10 days also eliminated symptoms but there was a return of symptoms on an 8-day course. Therefore subsequent treatment consisted of courses of 10 days prior to menstruation.

Fig. 13.5 Progressive shortening of initial course of progesterone. All symptoms were relieved on a 10-day course, but not on an 8-day course.

both the pregnancy and puerperium were normal there is a good chance that progesterone will no longer be required.

Duration

Women who have been incapacitated with premenstrual symptoms should be allowed at least three months on the lowest dosage and shortest course on which they are symptom-free before reducing the course still further. Then the course can be gradually reduced and stopped. When patients first stop progesterone after about three months the symptoms may return to their original pretreatment severity. If symptoms recur each time the dose is reduced or the course shortened the patient may need to continue indefinitely, or for a long period of time. At the menopause it is often possible to stop progesterone quite abruptly.

Unless their symptoms are very severe many women under 25 years of age are likely to need progesterone for only 6–9 months. Women over 40 years are likely to need progesterone therapy until the menopause. Factors which prolong the duration of treatment in those between 25 and 40 years include high parity, pre-eclampsia and postnatal depression.

Some patients who have been able to stop progesterone and remain symptom-free may find that at times of stress they have a recurrence of symptoms and then they will only need temporary progesterone treatment.

There does not seem to be any risk of developing tolerance to progesterone and there is no addiction.

Conception

Those anxious to conceive should start progesterone administration on day 16 or, if they are recording their basal temperature, the day after ovulation. They should then be advised to continue progesterone until the pregnancy has been confirmed.

Contraception

Patients with premenstrual syndrome usually have difficulty in tolerating the oestrogen-progestogen or the progestogen-only pill, probably because the progestogen lowers the plasma progesterone level (Table 3.3). If they have difficulty or strong objections to other contraceptive measures, after the optimum course of progesterone has been found, progesterone should be started on a low dose – for example, 100mg daily by suppository from day 8 until day 13, and the normal dose used from day 14 until the onset of menstruation. This is contraceptively safe but in a few women the early administration of progesterone in the follicular phase results in breakthrough bleeding on days 16–20. In this latter group the women may use norethisterone 0.5mg as in the progestogen-only pill, from day 5 until 14 and then use progesterone in the normal way.

The intrauterine device which slowly releases progesterone to the endometrium can be a useful form of contraception for sufferers of the premenstrual syndrome, but the small dose of progesterone has no therapeutic value. This is not available in Britain.

Individual tailoring

It will be appreciated that the course and dose of progesterone is individually tailored for each patient. This is not surprising in view of the innumerable presentations, differences in precise timing of symptoms variation in lengths of the menstrual cycle, desire for conception, or contraception and absorption variations.

Failure to respond

If a diabetic fails to respond to insulin, or a hypothyroid patient to thyroxine, the cause is either incorrect diagnosis or incorrect dosage. It is the same with premenstrual syndrome: if a patient fails to respond to progesterone one should check that the diagnosis is correct and ensure that the dosage has been increased to the limit.

Incorrect diagnosis

The failure of Sampson (1979) to differentiate between menstrual distress and premenstrual syndrome in her double-blind trials of progesterone and placebo inevitably led to the conclusion that progesterone was no better than placebo (see p. 27). Having had an opportunity to peruse her patients' questionnaires it became obvious that women with spasmodic dysmenorrhoea and endometriosis were included in her diagnosis of premenstrual syndrome, and it is well recognised that progesterone will not benefit patients with these conditions. In Chapters 3 and 4 great emphasis has been placed on the need to diagnose premenstrual syndrome carefully, for progesterone will benefit only premenstrual syndrome and not the many other menstrual disorders that are discussed in those chapters.

When faced with a patient with incapacitating symptoms, which she claims are related to menstruation, it is a great temptation to start progesterone treatment without a definitive menstrual record, especially in those who have travelled a considerable distance or have waited many months for appointment.

A business executive of 40 years brought a doctor's letter stating she had 'a clear history of premenstrual migraine'. She was first seen during menstruation and stated she had been incapacitated by migraine on six of the previous eight days, but she did not have a menstrual record. She was started on progesterone suppositories which brought no relief, but after two months it was clear from her menstrual chart and her completed attack forms that the symptoms were not related to menstruation. She did not have a phase free from migraine during the cycle and her migraine proved to be caused by certain foods in her diet.

There is of course no harm in a therapeutic trial so long as it is recognised as such, and provided that such women are not included in clinical trials and that the patient herself recognises that a diagnosis of premenstrual syndrome has not been made.

Incorrect dosage

If the menstrual record and history confirm the diagnosis of premenstrual syndrome, one is then justified in raising the daily injection dose to 100mg from ovulation until the onset of menstruation, and if necessary allowing the patient to supplement with up to 4×400mg suppositories each day before deciding that she has not responded to treatment. The rate and completeness of rectal and vaginal absorption vary: for some patients the effect of progesterone is too shortlived and they may need intramuscular injections.

An example of failure due to incorrect dosage is shown in the double-blind trials reported by Smith in which he gave 50mg progesterone injections on alternate days from days 19 to 26. As will be seen in Figs 14.1, 14.3 & 14.4 the duration of progesterone differs in each individual but a therapeutic dose never lasts longer than 48 hours; therefore, it would seem that failure in Smith's trial were due to giving progesterone in too low a dose, too late, after too long an interval and for too short a course. It is yet another example of a trial doomed to failure.

14

Progesterone suppositories and pessaries

Progesterone is a white crystalline powder which is dissolved in inert wax to form suppositories or pessaries, the same preparation being used for either the rectal or vaginal route. The wax has a low melting point, as several women have discovered when travelling in hot countries. Their shelf life is two years. Their great advantage is that of self-administration, and for this reason suppositories and pessaries are surprisingly well-accepted by most women, particularly if their symptoms are severe.

Nillius and Johansson studied the pattern of rectal absorption after giving 25mg and 100mg progesterone to two groups of women of fertile age during the follicular phase. Peak plasma concentrations of progesterone were obtained at 4–8 hours after administration, followed by a gradual decline. It should be noted that one of the subjects, who received 25mg, showed only an insignificant increase in plasma progesterone (Fig. 14.1).

One woman was studied by Nillius and Johansson during the follicular phase after rectal administration of 100mg progesterone at 24-hour intervals for five days, and they also obtained the plasma progesterone levels at 12 and 24 hours. They found it was not possible to maintain a stable elevated plasma level of progesterone with the dosage although there was a tendency to a cumulative effect during the five days of treatment. They noted that the rise and fall in plasma progesterone levels coincided with pronounced 'early pregnancy symptoms' such as nausea and depression (Fig. 14.2).

Nillius and Johansson also studied the plasma concentrations

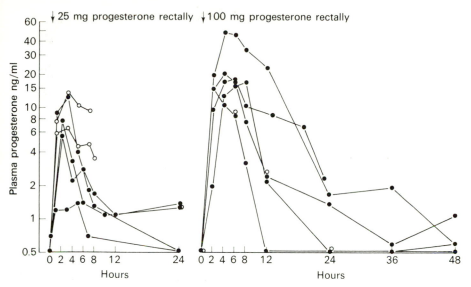

Fig. 14.1   Plasma levels of progesterone after rectal administration to two groups of six women in the follicular phase of the menstrual cycle. (From Nillius S.J., Johansson E.D.B. (1971). *Amer. J. Obs. Gynecol.;* **110**:4, 470.)

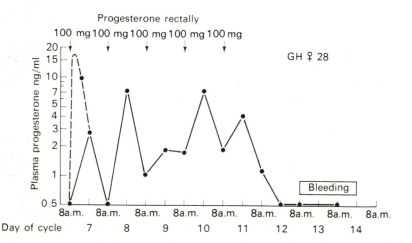

Fig. 14.2   Plasma levels of progesterone before, during and after five days of daily rectal administration of 100mg progesterone to a woman in the follicular phase of the menstrual cycle. (From Nillius S.J., Johansson E.D.B. (1971). *Amer. J. Obs. Gynecol.;* **710**:4, 470.)

of progesterone after vaginal administration of 100mg progesterone to six women of fertile age during the follicular phase. There was a rapid increase in plasma levels of progesterone reaching a peak within four hours and gradually falling during the following eight hours, although after 24 hours three of the women still had a plasma concentration of progesterone above the level normally found in the follicular phase of the menstrual cycle (Fig. 14.3).

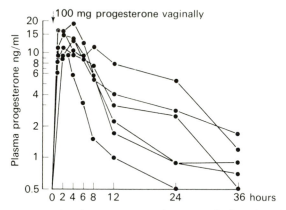

Fig. 14.3   Plasma levels of progesterone after vaginal administration of 100mg progesterone to six women in the follicular phase of the menstrual cycle. (From Nillius S.J., Johansson E.D.B. (1971). *Amer. J. Obs. Gynecol.*; **110**:4, 470.)

Clinical observation would support these findings of Nillius and Johansson as regards the short duration of action of rectal absorption, the discovery of some patients in whom there is poor rectal absorption, and the effect of the cumulative action which is manifested after several days' treatment. For this reason it is frequently necessary to administer suppositories and pessaries two to four times daily, and to start treatment five days before the expected onset of symptoms.

There is considerable individual variation in the absorption patterns and Nillius & Johansson estimated that it required about four times the injection dose to produce the same rise in plasma level of progesterone as that obtained by the rectal or vaginal route. Even so, the duration of action of a suppository or pessary is considerably shorter than the injection.

The absorption of progesterone also varies in different

individuals both in the peak levels reached and the time lapse before peak levels are attained. This may, in part, be related to the actual base used for the suppository.

Van der Meer and colleagues (1982) studied in three post-menopausal women and three male volunteers the absorption of two different types of fatty base, Witepsol H15 and Cyclogest (the age of the participants is not stated). Figures 14.4 and 14.5 show the different absorption levels at one, two and six hours. Among the three postmenopausal women, one test reached the highest level at one hour, another at two hours, and four at six hours, while among the men, one test reached the highest level at one hour and the other five at six hours. One of the men never reached the normal range of 30–60nmol/l expected in normal menstruating women in the luteal phase. It is much to be regretted that these studies were not performed on normal menstruating women in the follicular phase, and that the level of oestrogen in the postmenopausal women or the level of testosterone in the men were unknown, for these are all factors affecting progesterone absorption and SHBG levels (Dalton, M.E.).

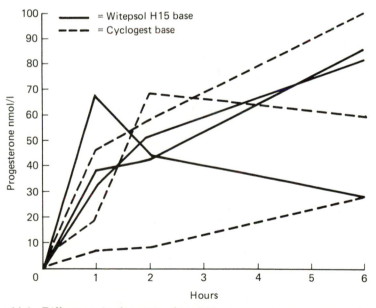

Fig. 14.4   Differences in absorption from 200mg progesterone suppositories in three postmenopausal women. (Compiled from data by Van der Meer Y. G. *et al.* (1982). *Pharm. Weekblad. Scient. Ed.*; **4**:135.)

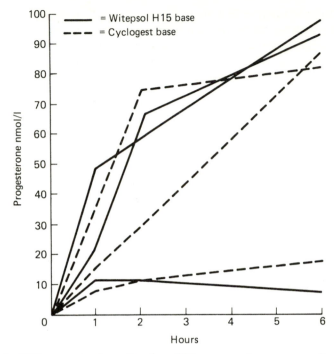

Fig. 14.5   Differences in absorption from 200mg progesterone suppositories in three male volunteers. (Compiled from data by Van der Meer Y.G. *et al.* (1982). *Pharm. Weekblad. Scient. Ed.*; **4**:135.)

In practice, suppositories and pessaries are interchangeable and it is left to the individual to decide on the route. There are cultural variations determining the choice, and some women use both routes alternately. With vaginal administration there is no effective sphincter to control the leakage of wax, so some women use this route at night when soiling underclothes is not such a problem, and use the rectal route in the morning. Others prefer the pessaries in the morning so as not to interfere with the habitual morning opening of the bowels. Patients should be advised that if they defaecate within an hour of the insertion of the suppository another one should be used.

Rectal use is also advised for women who are using a contraceptive diaphragm because the suppository base may affect the rubber used in the diaphragm. Regular users of progesterone are, however, contraceptively safe 24 hours after starting the course.

Permission is given to patients to use an extra suppository or pessary during the day if they feel the need, such as an impending migraine, sudden onset of tiredness, depression or irritability, or wheezing, and at times of stress. Patients soon learn their own requirements and the time interval which suits them best.

Some women have observed that if they use half a 400mg suppository instead of a whole 200mg the problem of wax leakage is decreased.

Dosage

The usual starting dose for a nulliparous woman is 400mg suppository daily, and for the parous woman 400mg twice daily from ovulation until menstruation. The optimum dose for 565 women seen in 1982 is shown in Table 14.1, with further statistics in Appendix. The low doses of 200mg × ½ or 200mg × 1 are used exclusively for contraception in those women with premenstrual syndrome who develop side effects with oral contraceptives. In Britain the 200mg suppository is the lowest dosage available, but 50mg is adequate for contraception.

Table 14.1

Dosage of progesterone administered

Suppositories daily	n=565 n	%
200mg × ½	17	3
200mg × 1	35	6
200mg × 2	7	1
400mg × 1	101	18
400mg × 2	192	34
400mg × 3	99	18
400mg × 4	30	5
400mg × 6	9	2
Injections		
50mg daily	2	0.4
100mg alternative days	3	0.5
100mg daily	45	8
Implant	25	4

Side effects
Anal soreness, diarrhoea and flatulence may occur with the suppositories. In cases of anal soreness the patient may be advised to use a bland ointment at the time of insertion. After using pessaries patients may complain of vaginal discharge, which is the leakage of the inert wax.

Contraindications
Suppositories should be avoided in women with a history of colitis and faecal incontinence. Pessaries are contraindicated in those with vaginal infection, especially moniliasis, and in those with recurrent cystitis.

Comparison of effectiveness of injections with suppositories and pessaries
Controlled trials into the prophylactic value of progesterone injection in pre-eclampsia (Dalton, 1962) were later repeated using the same protocol but with suppositories or pessaries instead. The dosage used was the lowest which would control the pregnancy symptoms in each individual. The results of the trials showed a remarkable similarity in effectiveness whether progesterone injections were used or suppositories (Table 14.2) (see Chapter 20).

Table 14.2

Comparisons of progesterone injections and suppositories or pessaries

| | Progesterone | | Controls | |
	Injections	Suppositories or pessaries	Injections	Suppositories or pessaries
Number in group	62	80	66	88
	%	%	%	%
Pre-eclampsia	3*	3*	11	11
BP over 140/90	11*	11	20	19
Oedema	4*	6*	17	18
Proteinuria	2	—*	7	7

*=Probability<0.05

15

Progesterone injections

Progesterone is insoluble in water but soluble in alcohol, arachis oil, chloroform and ether. The BP preparation of progesterone is dissolved in ethyloleate. Occasionally solid matter separates out on prolonged standing in the cold; should this occur it may be dissolved by slowly heating the ampoule.

Indications for progesterone injection

1. Failure to respond to suppositories or pessaries.
2. Suppositories and pessaries are contraindicated or/and disliked by the patient, or unobtainable.
3. Hospital patients.
4. Those requiring daily supervision by a nurse, as where there is a risk of suicide, battering or alcoholic bout.

Duration of action

Nillius and Johansson studied eight menstruating women in the follicular phase of the cycle and four postmenopausal women after intramuscular injection of 100mg progesterone and found that a peak level was usually obtained within eight hours, and raised levels persisted for up to 48 hours in most subjects (Fig. 15.1).

They also found the rise in plasma progesterone proportional to the dose given. One woman volunteered for five experiments during a one-year period and it was possible to determine the effectiveness of various doses and routes of administration (Fig. 15.2).

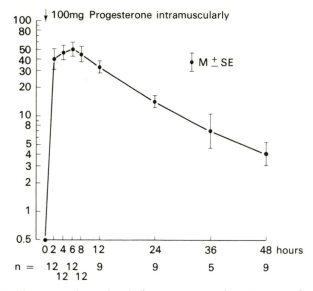

Fig. 15.1   The mean plasma level of progesterone after intramuscular administration of 100mg progesterone to eight women in the follicular phase of
the menstrual cycle and four postmenopausal women. (From Nillius
S.J., Johansson E.D.B. (1971). *Amer. J. Obs. Gynecol*; **110**:4, 470.)

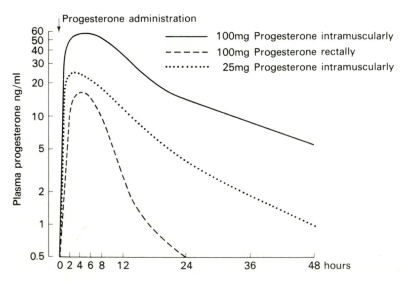

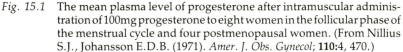

Fig. 15.2   Plasma progesterone levels following intramuscular injections and
rectal administration. (From Nillius S.J., Johansson E.D.B. (1971). *Acta
Endocrin.*; **1**:68; **4**:17–20.)

The studies of Nillius and Johansson confirm the clinical observation that progesterone injections need to be given daily or at least on alternate days. Some women, particularly those receiving treatment for the relief of pregnancy symptoms, notice that if injections are given on alternate days they have alternate symptomatic and symptom free days.

Administration

Progesterone injections require a site where there are ample fat cells so that a depot of progesterone can be formed for the release into the blood. The gluteal muscles have fat cells between the muscle fibres, which act in this way – hence progesterone injections are best given deep into the buttock rather than the thigh or deltoid area. A 1½ inch (3.8cm) needle should be used, as too superficial an injection may cause soreness and possible urticaria. It is wise to use one needle for drawing up the solution and another for injections, to avoid infiltration of the dermis by progesterone or solvent on the surface of the needle.

As will be seen in Fig. 15.3 there is an ample injection area in the buttocks and nurses should be instructed to inject into the buttocks wherever there is a two-inch pinch of flesh. They should also avoid injecting into an area that is either hot or hard. The raised temperature of the skin can be recognised by gently passing the back of a hand over the buttock.

The soreness that may result from injection appears to be more the property of the solvent than the active ingredient, for during controlled trials when patients were injected at random with either progesterone or the solvent only, it was found that as many complaints of soreness at the injection site arose from those receiving the solvent alone as from those receiving progesterone (Dalton, 1962).

Initially, the injections may be given by the practice, district or factory nurse, but with suitable instruction most patients soon learn the art of giving their own injections. Failing this, the husbands may be ready to learn the technique. The use of an injection gun gives many patients the necessary initial confidence for self-injection. For women at risk during the premenstruum the daily visit of a nurse to give the injection is a valuable form of silent supervision.

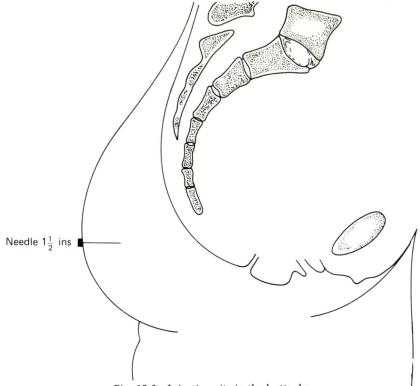

Needle $1\frac{1}{2}$ ins

Fig. 15.3   Injection site in the buttocks.

Dosage

Progesterone injections are available in ampoules of 25mg, 50mg and 100mg. In the non-pregnant woman it is rarely necessary to exceed 100mg daily, but during pregnancy, when the progesterone levels are considerably raised, doses of 100mg may be given three times daily for not more than seven days.

After an intramuscular injection some women experience the characteristic taste of progesterone within three minutes of injection. This is due to the rapid metabolism, with some of the metabolites being excreted via the lungs. These women are always the ones who obtain positive benefit from progesterone and are usually those who require daily injections (Dalton, 1964).

Side effects

Some women develop an abscess after several months or years of progesterone injections. It is common among those who, giving their own injections, repeatedly use the same site, or inject using too short a needle. The abscess is caused by unabsorbed oil, it is deep-seated and sterile; however, it may remain unresolved and need incision and drainage. If the buttock is hot or inflamed, injections should not be given; suppositories or pessaries must be used as alternatives. As it is a sterile abscess antibiotics are unnecessary.

16

Progesterone implantation

Compressed pellets of pure progesterone are obtainable in doses of 100mg and 200mg and may be implanted in the fat of the anterior abdominal wall to eliminate the need for too frequent injections, suppositories or pessaries.

An implant gives a continuous supply of progesterone, whereas normally a menstruating woman would have an appreciable level of blood progesterone only during the luteal phase. It is therefore not surprising that in some women a progesterone implant may disrupt the normal cyclical pattern with irregular scanty prolonged bleeding for up to three weeks followed by spells of amenorrhoea which may last up to six months, while in other women menstruation continues at its normal regular pattern.

Extrusion of pellet

At times when the progesterone level would normally be raised in the luteal phase the site of the implant may often become sore or inflamed, suggesting that extra blood is reaching the site to correct the low progesterone blood level. If this is not corrected the inflammation develops and the pellet may be extruded, either through the site of insertion or directly through the skin above where the pellet lay. Women should be advised that if the site becomes sore or red they should supplement their progesterone supply by using suppositories 400mg three times daily or injections of 100mg daily for five consecutive days or until the site has normalised.

Extrusions of one or more pellets are likely to occur if given into the fascia lata or thigh muscles where there are few fat cells, or if given to a patient already depleted of progesterone. Extrusions have been known to occur as soon as two weeks or as late as 16 months after implantation, but extrusions are rare in pregnancy.

Indications for implantation

1. Women who have had complete relief of symptoms on progesterone injections, suppositories or pessaries.
2. Those still having cyclical symptoms after the menopause or hysterectomy.
3. Erratic users of progesterone, such as the feckless alcoholics.

One patient living in Italy calculated that the cost of an annual implant plus the air fare from Rome to London was cheaper than the cost of daily suppositories.

Contraindications

1. Those wishing to conceive within 12 months. A progesterone implant inhibits ovulation for many months.
2. Those unduly concerned by irregular menstruation, scanty loss or spells of amenorrhoea which may last about six months.
3. Those whose progesterone requirement is too high – that is, above 75mg injection daily or 400mg three times a day by suppository or pessary.

Preliminary precautions

To diminish the possibility of extrusion of the pellets one should ensure that the patient has had regular progesterone during the five days immediately before implantation, and that the woman is either still menstruating or in the immediate postmenstruum.

Dosage

The usual dose for a non-pregnant woman is 5–16 pellets of 100mg. As several pellets are required, a progesterone implant is not as easy to perform as an oestrogen implant.

Duration

The duration of action of an implant may vary between 3 and 12 months. Some patients find that repeated implants all have the same duration of action, while in others it may vary for no obvious reason.

An analysis of effectiveness

An analysis of the effectiveness of 77 progesterone implants given to 71 patients with premenstrual syndrome failed to reveal any significant factor relating to the duration of effectiveness. In particular it did not appear to be related to the following:

1. Type or timing of symptoms within the menstrual cycle.
2. Time in the cycle at which the implantation was performed.
3. Presence or absence of bleeding or bruising at the implant site.
4. Batch number of progesterone pellets used.
5. Tendency to extrusion.
6. Depth of abdominal fat.
7. Presence or absence of pain at the implant site.
8. Dose of progesterone used in the implant.

The end of the effectiveness of an implant is usually very gradual with a return of tension symptoms before the somatic symptoms of migraine, epilepsy or asthma return. Frequently it is the husband who first notices, by his wife's bad temper, that the time for further treatment has come.

Requirements for implantation

1. Pellets of progesterone (the usual dose is 5–16 pellets ×100mg).
2. Local anaesthetic, e.g. 5ml 2% lignocaine.
3. Scalpel.
4. Wide trocar and cannula. (The trocar and cannula used for an oestrogen implant has too small a bore.)
5. Suture material.
6. Skin-marking pencil.

Method

1. Choose a site in the iliac fossa and mark the skin radially 5mm from the proposed incision to show where the pellets are to be implanted and to ensure that the local anaesthetic penetrates these areas (Fig. 16.1).
2. Anaesthetise the area using 5ml 2% lignocaine.

3. Under local anaesthetic make a 1cm incision into the skin of the anterior abdominal wall.
4. Insert cannula to the full extent, deep into the fat and close to the abdominal muscle layer, pointing in the direction of one of the points marked on the skin.
5. Place one or two 100mg progesterone implant pellets into the cannula and push home with trocar to the full extent. If more than six pellets are being used, two pellets may be embedded at the same site at the same time.
6. Remove trocar and cannula and reinsert in the same cut pointing in a different direction, and insert more pellets.
7. Suture the incision with one absorbable suture.

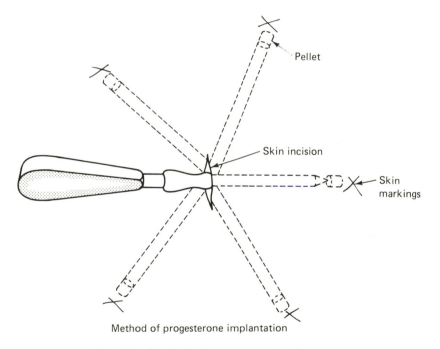

Method of progesterone implantation

Fig. 16.1   Method of progesterone implantation.

After each implantation the patient should be advised that if the site becomes red or inflamed she should have progesterone injections 100mg daily or suppositories 400mg three times daily for five consecutive days to prevent any possibility of an extrusion of a pellet. If the suture has not been absorbed within five days it should be removed.

Side effects

Subsequently there may be some tenderness and bruising for a few days in slim patients, but the obese are usually surprisingly free from pain. The following week the pellets may be felt as round masses or, as one patient described it, 'like a sack of new potatoes'.

Insomnia and restless energy may be noted for the first few days, and it may be necessary to give mild sedation, but this requirement rarely lasts long.

17

Clinical studies

A survey of medical publications on premenstrual syndrome and progesterone therapy suggests that these two areas are extraordinarily difficult ones for critical scientific studies because they present innumerable problems for the unwary investigator. There is the crucial importance of the definition and diagnosis, discussed fully in Chapters 2 and 3; the need to differentiate between premenstrual symptoms and premenstrual syndrome; the vital differentiation of premenstrual syndrome from menstrual distress, considered in Chapter 4; the difference between progesterone and progestogens (Chapter 10) but there will still remain a multiplicity of other complications that are seldom recognised and not very easily overcome.

The following are some of the other problems that may cause difficulty and need to be taken into account.

Variations in the length of the menstrual cycle
Biology students are taught the changes in the menstrual cycle using a model of 28 days, but among women there is an amazing diversity with the normal range being between 21 and 35 days, but cycles can vary by up to four days month by month and still be accepted as normal. This normal variation needs to be recognised when considering any special investigation, such as a blood test, weighing, or filling in a questionnaire which requires to be done on a specific day. The selection of day 28 for such a procedure could result in a large proportion of the sample not being tested because the cycle was shorter than 28 days. Similarly, it cannot be assumed that ovulation is precisely on day 14, which could be in

the luteal phase in women with a short cycle or the follicular phase in those with long cycles. One must recognise that most women claim to have a 28-day cycle, so at the initial interview a useful test question is 'Which day of the week does menstruation start?' If there is a precise 28-day cycle it will always start on the same day of the week and will be only one day early, by date, year by year or two days in a leap year. Others will claim it always starts on the same date of each month, imagining that their menstrual controlling centre makes allowances for 28 days in February. Coppen and Kessel in a survey of 500 women in south London in 1963 noted that 16% did not know the date of their next menstruation. One wonders if this has improved over the years with the attention given to the hazards of the menstrual cycle. Women with cycles outside the range of 21–35 days may need to be excluded because there is a strong possibility that their cycles are anovular; even so, it must not be forgotten that premenstrual syndrome can and does occur in anovular cycles.

Variations in menstrual flow

Normal menstruation may last from two to eight days, although in teenagers it tends to last longer and with a lighter loss. The pattern of flow varies from a heavy initial flow for two or three days followed by a slight loss till the end of menstruation, to the presence of a scanty initial loss for a few days before the full menstrual flow (see Fig. 5.1). Those who have an intact intra-uterine device may have a few days of premenstrual spotting before and after the full menstruation. It is usual for premenstrual syndrome to ease with the full menstrual flow, which explains why some women still have symptoms during the first few days of menstruation. The problem this poses for investigators is which day should be recorded as the first day of menstruation? The first day of slight loss? When the loss becomes normal? Or when the flow is heavy?

Age

It must be appreciated that premenstrual syndrome increases in incidence and in severity with age. On the other hand, spasmodic dysmenorrhoea is common in teenagers and up to 25 years of age and yet many investigators of premenstrual syndrome seek volunteers for their studies from among young nurses and students, the very age group that is high in spasmodic dysmenorrhoea and low in premenstrual syndrome.

Parity

Premenstrual syndrome increases with parity, especially when the pregnancies have been complicated by pre-eclampsia or post-natal depression (Tables 8.3 & 27.11). Investigators too often fail to make allowances for parity or fail to mention the incidence of these complications.

Hormone levels

Women who have recently received hormone treatment or oral contraceptives ought to be excluded, as should those who have had bilateral tubal ligations, for all these factors alter the normal hormone levels (Radwanska *et al.*).

Stress

An individual's menstrual pattern may be altered by stress, which may either lengthen or shorten the cycle or the duration of menstruation. It can increase any premenstrual or menstrual symptoms. In studies using students and lasting for over a month it is important to include information on the times of examinations and vacations to give some indication of how many volunteers were under stress during the time of the investigation.

Severity of symptoms

Premenstrual syndrome varies in severity from mild, hardly noticeable symptoms to life-threatening conditions. Studying only the mild presentations in the general population will not necessarily help a greater understanding of severe symptomatology.

   Clare (1982) administered self-rating questionnaires to identify premenstrual complainers in a healthy population, and having divided them into psychiatrically healthy and psychiatrically ill premenstrual complainers, drew conclusions on the degree of neuroticism and anxiety traits of premenstrual syndrome sufferers. Studies of mild symptoms in women who have not sought medical help must be recognised as different from studies in women with severe symptoms requiring help. Surveys of this type are as irrelevant to the elucidation of the aetiology or treatment of premenstrual syndrome as a similar population study of diarrhoea sufferers would be in investigating aetiological or therapeutic factors in ulcerative colitis or Crohn's disease.

Ethnic background

Janiger (p. 97) has shown the difference in severity of premenstrual symptoms in the various ethnic groups, reminding the investigator that this is yet another factor to be noted in the sample and to be considered in the findings.

General health

Subjects for clinical studies into premenstrual syndrome are usually required to be of good general health and free from medication, which automatically excludes those on anticonvulsants, antidepressants and bronchial dilators, yet these may be patients suffering from the very disease which is being studied.

Contraception

A full knowledge of the subject's hopes or fears regarding a possible pregnancy need to be known in advance when a self-rating daily questionnaire is being completed. If menstruation is delayed it will bring happiness to those hoping to conceive but anxiety to those with inadequate contraception. Oral contraception and sterilisation will interfere with hormonal studies. An intrauterine device frequently alters the length of the cycle and duration of loss.

Selection of subjects

The greatest problem comes in the selection of subjects for double-blind controlled therapeutic trials, because it is ethically wrong to include those in danger of harming themselves or others, and this automatically excludes those at risk of an epileptic attack, acute self-destructive acts, asthmatic attacks, suicide, homicide, violence, criminal damage, or alcoholic bouts. Women with moderate premenstrual syndrome who have completed a three-month chart are usually at the end of their tether and demand treatment; they are no longer ready to accept the possibility of receiving placebo treatment. On the other hand, those with only mild premenstrual syndrome do not warrant hormone treatment and can be managed by simpler means (Chapter 11). In any case, their response to progesterone will not necessarily compare with that of sufferers with moderate or severe premenstrual syndrome. This difficulty can be partly overcome by treating the patients first and then, when they have had several months completely free of premenstrual syndrome, asking them to volunteer for a month's trial of some other drug (Dalton, 1959 and 1976) or a placebo. The women then know that their suffering can be relieved and have permission to return to effective treatment should they consider it to be necessary.

Selection of controls

Controls need to be of the same age, parity, social class, health, intelligence and ethnic group as the subjects suffering from premenstrual syndrome. A curious selection of subjects and controls are to be found in some studies. A few examples are given below.

Biased selection of subjects and controls occurred when limiting the studies to women attending an infertility clinic (Benedek-Jaszman and Hearn-Sturtevant, 1976).

The use of lithium in premenstrual syndrome was tested on 19 patients in hospital including five with schizophrenia, four neurotics and three psychotics (Singer *et al.*, 1974).

A study of minor psychiatric and physical symptoms in premenstrual syndrome selected seven control women who had undergone a hysterectomy (Beaumont *et al.*, 1975).

Abraham (1982) chose controls from those who suffered 'only minor premenstrual symptoms'.

An appeal on commercial radio asked for volunteers for premenstrual syndrome trials in London. The authors stated, in the report of their finding, that a telephone conversation ensured that the volunteers all had premenstrual complaints, but after one month's charting of symptoms only three had premenstrual symptoms alone, 34 had premenstrual and menstrual symptoms (Wood and Jakubowicz, 1980).

None of these trials are acceptable, because of their biased selection.

Moos menstrual distress questionnaire

The failure to diagnose premenstrual syndrome from questionnaires has already been discussed (pp. 26–28). A further fault which must be mentioned is the limitation of the use of the questionnaire from day 21 until menstruation, such as occurred in the trials of bromocriptine in premenstrual syndrome by Elser *et al.* (1980).

This will guarantee an absence of recorded symptoms in the postmenstruum.

Like must be compared with like

In eliciting the effect of progesterone, subjects need to be normally menstruating women, yet Oelkers *et al.* (1974) studied the effect on 20 male medical students. Nor can it be assumed that the metabolism of progesterone in normal menstruating women is the same as that found in women who experienced a normal menopause two to five years previously (Whitehead *et al.*, 1980).

Species differences

Menstruation in humans is not the same as oestrus in animals. The function of progesterone varies among the species.

Double diagnosis

Women who already have a known disease are unsuitable for any investigations into premenstrual syndrome. Day (1979) reported three patients with irritability and depression as their main premenstrual symptoms and who were treated with danazol, but he stated that two of them also had proven endometriosis. Osborn (1981) proposed studying premenstrual tension in women who were awaiting simple hysterectomy for benign menorrhagia by first investigating them while on the waiting list and then again at six months postoperatively, when the premenstruum would be identified by serial progesterone levels.

Effect of medication on following cycle

If the aetiological hypothesis proposed in Chapter 9 has any validity, in double-blind controlled trials consideration must be given to the carryover or residual effects of the active drug in the month after its administration. A good crossover design suggested by Sampson and Prescott (1981) would seem of value. For sequences of four cycles with active (A) and placebo (P) treatment is APPA, AAPP, PAAP, and PPAA, in which the second A is compared with the second P or the initial A if A was used first.

Reporting of results

The problems of clinical studies do not end with the selection of subjects and controls. Perusal of the completed paper and checking of the statistical analysis are absolutely essential. Kerr and his co-workers (1980) cleverly overcame the problem of a high placebo response by adding the 51% improvement noted during active and placebo treatment to the 21% noted by the women when only on the active treatment with dydrogesterone – and so they claimed that 72% of patients improved on treatment with dydrogesterone.

Progesterone studies

Little reference is made in medical literature to the progesterone studies that have already been carried out, thus giving the impression that there has been no work on this subject. Nevertheless, work on premenstrual syndrome and progesterone has been continuing for the last 35 years and statistics on the subject are to be found in the text and the appendix.

Progesterone had already been successfully used by Gray in 1941, Puech in 1942 and Albeaus-Fernet and Loublie in 1946 before the first report appeared in British medical literature by Greene and Dalton in 1953 in the *British Medical Journal*. That report detailed 86 women suffering from premenstrual syndrome of whom 83.5% become symptom-free and 6.6% improved with progesterone injections while only 47.9% became symptom-free and 17.4% improved with oral ethisterone.

The value of progesterone injections for the relief of pregnancy symptoms and the prevention of pre-eclampsia was reported in the *British Medical Journal* in 1957. Of 136 women, who had all received complete relief from progesterone injections, only 59.8% obtained relief from oral ethisterone (Chapter 20) (Dalton, 1957).

A comparative trial of 58 patients suffering from premenstrual syndrome, all of whom had complete symptomatic relief from progesterone injections and who volunteered for trials of oral progestogens, was reported in the *British Medical Journal* in 1959. There was a 36% benefit from ethisterone, 42% from dimethisterone and 40% from norethisterone, but within three months all the volunteers opted to return to progesterone injections which they knew brought them full symptomatic relief (Dalton, 1959).

In 1962 controlled trials into the prophylactic value of progesterone in the treatment of pre-eclampsia showed that giving progesterone injections to women with pregnancy symptoms in the second trimester of pregnancy onwards prevented the development of pre-eclampsia. The symptomatic treatment group and the progesterone treatment group were allocated by random selection during the second trimester. These trials showed that only 3.7% of the progesterone-treated group developed pre-eclampsia compared with 10.6% of the symptomatic group. The same protocol was used in trials from 1973 to 1974 when progesterone suppositories were used instead of progesterone injections; the results were similar, with 3% of the progesterone-treated groups developing pre-eclampsia compared with 11% of the symptomatic group (Table 14.2 & Chapter 20) (Dalton, 1962).

In 1968 the first report of the advantages of antenatal progesterone on intelligence appeared, followed in 1976 by the folow-up of the children at 18–20 years. Children whose mothers had received antenatal progesterone were compared with the next-born child in the labour ward register, whose mother had a normal pregnancy and delivery. The children of the progesterone-treated mothers were shown to have advanced development at one year, higher academic standards at 9–10 years, better educational attainments at school-leaving age with a higher proportion of university entrants. The best academic results were obtained by the children whose mothers received over 5gm antenatal progesterone; where treatment began before the 16th week of pregnancy and whose treatment continued for longer than eight weeks (see pp. 133–139).

In 1973 the use of progesterone suppositories and pessaries in the treatment of menstrual migraine was published in the American journal *Headache*.

In 1975 12 of my patients suffering from severe premenstrual syndrome – and fully controlled on progesterone suppositories – volunteered for comparative trials with bromocriptine, reported at the symposium on bromocriptine at the Royal College of Physicians, London. After the first month eight voted to return to progesterone and by the fourth month they were all back on their usual progesterone medication.

It is agreed that the ideal is to be able to report double-blind controlled trials of progesterone in patients with severe premenstrual syndrome, but the many problems of such clinical studies have already been discussed.

Haskett *et al.* (1979) in a study into severe premenstrual tension, rejected 80% of 254 volunteers and then, in their conclusions, had to accept that 40% of the 42 women selected were unsuitable for the study. It should be noted that rejection was on interview only, for they had no clinical examination.

Among the many bizarre psychological studies of premenstrual syndrome, that of Foresti *et al.* (1981) must take the prize, for they set out to study premenstrual syndrome and its personality traits in 110 women in the eighth month of their pregnancy. Surely even psychotherapists should know that there is no menstruation during pregnancy and that the woman's highest blood progesterone level occurs during late pregnancy.

18

Adjustment of menstruation

The deleterious effects of the premenstrual syndrome are described in Chapters 5 and 6. The time of risk is invariably the paramenstruum with relative freedom from these disturbances during other phases of the cycle and, indeed, an increased sense of wellbeing in the postmenstruum. The extent to which these paramenstrual influences have a prejudicial effect on the sufferer is a very individual matter. The adjustment of menstruation to avoid those deleterious effects at times when the patient requires to be at the peak of her abilities can be fully justified.

With our greater understanding of the menstrual hormones, adjustment of menstruation is now a practical proposition, and in fact this is exactly what happens when a woman goes on the oestrogen-progestogen contraceptive pill. Nevertheless, the mere postponement of menstruation, which allows a prolongation of the incapacitating premenstrual symptoms, is of no value.

It must be emphasised that not all women are handicapped by menstruation. There are those who have anovular cycles, following a period of amenorrhoea, and these women are usually remarkably free from paramenstrual symptoms.

Adjustment of menstruation has been requested by students, sportswomen and actresses in respect of specific occasions such as examination, interviews, competitions or performances. The event may last only a single day or be continuous over a period of three or more weeks. It may be a request purely for social convenience as for a wedding, or a holiday jet flight. A prerequisite to the adjustment of menstruation is an accurate menstrual chart with a known date of the event on which menstruation is to be avoided. In this respect there is a vital difference between a cycle of 28 days and one of 31 days, for after an interval of only a couple of cycles there would be a six-day difference in regard to the event. All too often the woman announces she has a regular cycle of 28 days.

It is also useful to have some idea of the phase in the cycle for her best performances, which again varies individually. It is often best between days 9–12 and 17–21, but some sportswomen are surprised to find that they perform best during their aggressive premenstrual phase. Students whose essays are marked weekly, and sportswomen who do a daily time check in training, may be able to give these particulars with accuracy. Figure 18.1 shows the dates of good and poor performances during the training programme of a sportswoman.

The drugs available to alter menstruation are oestrogens, progestogens, and progesterone. Any one of these, if given for a few days after ovulation and then stopped, may be expected to cause menstruation or withdrawal bleeding within 48 hours of cessation.

Oestrogens

Oestrogens are of value in the teenager who has immature sexual development or who suffers from spasmodic dysmenorrhoea. The side effects of oestrogen may be nausea, headache, weight gain and depression. Oestrogen may be conveniently given as ethinyloestradiol in doses of 10–50mg daily, or may be given with a progestogen as in the oestrogen-progestogen contraceptive pill.

Progestogens

Progestogens are useful for those with irregular and anovular menstruation. The 19 norsteroids are best, used in a dose of 5mg or as an oral progestogen-only contraceptive pill.

Progesterone

Progesterone is best for those with premenstrual syndrome, congestive dysmenorrhoea or with a tendency to suffer from bloatedness, weight gain, headaches or mood swings.

Method

The easiest cycles to adjust are those of women who are already on oral contraceptives, for the course can easily be extended or

	Jan.	Feb.	Mar.	Apr.
1				
2		✓		✓
3				
4				
5	✓			
6		✓		
7		✓		
8				
9			✓	
10				
11				
12			✓	
13			✓	
14	✳			
15	✳			✓
16	M ✳			✓
17	M			
18	M			
19	M	✳		
20	M	✳		
21		M		
22		M		
23		M	✳M	✳
24	✓	M	M	✳
25	✓		M	M
26			M	M
27			M	M
28			M	M
29				M
30			✓	
31				
Total				

Fig. 18.1 Performance and menstruation. (From Williams J.G.P., Sperryn P.N. (1976). *Sports Medicine*. London, E. Arnold.)

contracted and the time of menstruation reliably predicted. Furthermore, these women already know how soon bleeding starts after they have taken their last pill.

Ideally, if one is adjusting for a specific event it is best to adjust the cycles in the months beforehand so that no medication need be given in the month of the event. Figure 18.2 shows the chart of a sportswoman who had noted poor performances in the late premenstruum and early menstruation from February to April, her best performances were achieved in the postmenstruum. The cycle in May was shortened to 21 days by giving an oestrogen-progestogen pill from days 5 to 19. The next two menstruations occurred at their normal interval, allowing the woman to perform during her optimum phase of the postmenstruum.

	Jan.	Feb.	Mar.	Apr.	May	Jun.	Jul.
1					:		M
2					:		M
3					:	M	M
4					↓	M	
5						M	
6					M	M	
7					M		
8					M		
9							C
10							
11							
12				M			
13				M			
14				M			
15			M	M			
16		M	M	↑			
17		M	M	:			
18	M	M		:			
19	M	M		:			
20	M			:			
21	M			:			
22				:			
23				:			
24				:			
25				:			
26				:			
27				:			
28				:			
29				:			
30				:			
31							
Total							

The menstrual cycle in May was shortened. Normal menstruation occurred in June and July. M, menstruation; C, competition; ↑, treatment started; ↓, treatment stopped.

Fig. 18.2 Adjusting menstruation in a woman with a regular cycle. (From Williams J.G.P., Sperryn P.N. (1976). *Sports Medicine*. London, E. Arnold.)

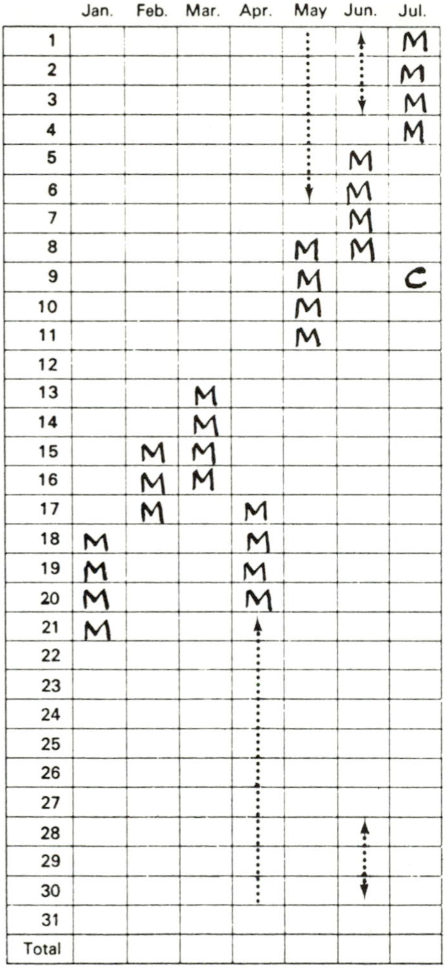

	Jan.	Feb.	Mar.	Apr.	May	Jun.	Jul.
1					⋮	↑	M
2					⋮	⋮	M
3					⋮	↓	M
4					⋮		M
5					⋮	M	
6					↑	M	
7						M	
8					M	M	
9					M		C
10					M		
11					M		
12							
13			M				
14			M				
15		M	M				
16		M	M				
17		M		M			
18	M			M			
19	M			M			
20	M			M			
21	M			↑			
22				⋮			
23				⋮			
24				⋮			
25				⋮			
26				⋮			
27				⋮			
28				⋮		↑	
29				⋮		⋮	
30				⋮		↓	
31							
Total							

Cycle length varies from 26 to 35 days. The menstrual cycle in May was shortened to 21 days. The June and July cycles were regularized with short 3-day courses of treatment. M, menstruation; C, competition; ↑, treatment started; ↓, treatment stopped.

Fig. 18.3   Adjusting menstruation in a woman with an irregular cycle. (From Williams J.G.P., Sperryn P.N. (1976). *Sports Medicine*. London, E. Arnold.)

	Jan.	Feb.	Mar.	Apr.	May	Jun.	Jul.
1							
2							
3							
4							
5							
6							
7						M	
8			M		M	M	
9			M	M	M	M	C
10			M	M	M	M	
11			M	M	M	M	
12			M	M	M	M	M
13			M	M	M	M	M
14			M	M	M	M	M
15				M			M
16							M
17							M
18							M
19							
20							
21							
22							
23							
24							
25							
26							
27							
28							
29							
30							
31							
Total							

Late consultation only 9 days before event, treated with progesterone.
Although progestogens will delay menstruation they will not prevent
premenstrual deterioration of performance. M, menstruation;
C, competition; ↟, treatment started; ⸪, treatment stopped.

Fig. 18.4 Late adjustment of menstruation. (From Williams J.G.P., Sperryn P.N. (1976). *Sports Medicine*. London, E. Arnold.)

On the other hand, the sportswoman whose chart is shown in Fig. 18.3 also had her poorest performances in the premenstruum, but had an irregular cycle varying from 26 to 35 days. The menstrual cycle was shortened in May to 21 days by giving an oestrogen-progestogen pill from days 5–19; but to ensure against the possibility of a long cycle in June or July a three-day course of the pill was also given on days 24–26 in June.

Inevitably, one is also consulted by those who attend too late to adjust their cycle properly. The candidate in Fig. 18.4 attended only nine days before the competition, which did not provide enough time in which to give the minimum of a three-day course of medication, to allow 48 hours for bleeding to occur and to have completed menstruation before the competition. So instead she was given a nine-day course of progesterone suppositories 400mg to use each morning until after the competition; this prevented premenstrual deterioration and postponed menstruation.

If it is desired to shorten the cycle by only two or three days or if menstruation is already overdue then medication need be given for only three days to be successful. If it is desired to shorten the cycle to 16 days, however, medication needs to be given continuously from day 5 until day 14. Progestogens may be given in this case, even to sufferers of the premenstrual syndrome, because there is no risk that they will reduce the blood progesterone level, which is absent during the follicular phase.

There may be a demand for a longer suppression of menstruation, as with an actress who may have a continuous programme of events for a few months. In this case oestrogens, progestogens, or progesterone may be used continuously, and although there may be the occasional breakthrough bleeding this is usually scanty, free from symptoms and does not affect performance. The dose should be the lowest compatible with suppression for each individual, and this can often be lowered at monthly intervals. Sufferers from spasmodic dysmenorrhoea, in particular, will benefit from such a regimen and may be free from dysmenorrhoea when it is decided to resume normal menstruation. It is now recognised that the contraceptive pill can be used continuously for three of four months but not, of course, by sufferers of premenstrual syndrome.

19

Dysmenorrhoea

Women who complain of pain with menstruation, and in whom a full physical and gynaecological examination reveals no abnormality, can be divided into two types:

1. *Spasmodic dysmenorrhoea*, sometimes called idiopathic dysmenorrhoea.
2. *Congestive dysmenorrhoea*, more accurately called premenstrual syndrome. In this group pain is a prominent symptom of their premenstrual syndrome and increases in intensity until the onset of the full menstrual flow.

Kessel and Coppen (1963), in their survey, discussed in Chapter 6, conclude: 'Pain was worst on the first day of the period. The other symptoms which tended to occur in the same woman were worst premenstrually. Thus there are two very common, but distinct entities – the premenstrual syndrome and dysmenorrhoea.' The time, relative to menstruation, when the various symptoms were said to be worst is shown in Fig. 19.1.

There is little difficulty in the differential diagnosis.

Spasmodic dysmenorrhoea is usually acute, with colicky pains occurring at intervals of about 20 minutes, and the girl is often to be found rolling herself into a ball to obtain ease, probably with a hot water bottle on her abdomen. The pain is limited to the area of the uterine and ovarian nerve distribution, being felt in the pelvic area, the back and possibly the inner sides of the thighs. It resembles labour pains, and occasionally it may be severe enough to cause reflex vomiting or fainting. The predominant mood is one of anxiety and fear.

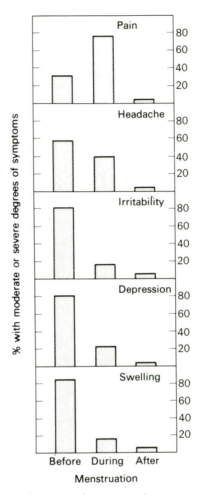

Fig. 19.1   Time of menstrual symptoms in a survey of 500 women.

Many sufferers of *premenstrual syndrome,* in contrast to spas-modic dysmenorrhoea, experience no pain with menstruation, and comment on the relief of their other symptoms when menstruation starts. If there is pain, however, it is a continuous, heavy dragging pain or bloatedness in the lower abdomen, increasing in severity during the premenstrual days to reach its zenith on the first day of menstruation. It may be accompanied by pains in other parts of the body, such as the breasts, head, back, and generalised pains in the joints and muscles, all characteristically accompanied by mood changes, with depression, irritability and lethargy (Fig. 19.2).

Because spasmodic dysmenorrhoea is related to ovular cycles, pain does not accompany the first anovular cycles but usually starts a couple of years after the menarche. The first attack of

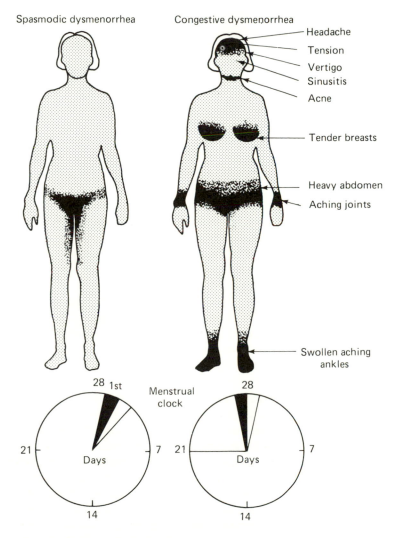

Fig. 19.2   Time and site of symptoms of dysmenorrhoea. (From Dalton K. (1969). *The Menstrual Cycle*. Penguin Books.)

dysmenorrhoea may be quite acute and unexpected owing to the previous pain-free menstruations. These painful menstruations may then alternate with painless menstruation for about six months until they settle down into regular ovular cycles. The premenstrual syndrome, in contrast, is present in both ovular and anovular cycles, and indeed the regular occurrence of abdominal pain and other premenstrual symptoms may be charted even before the first menstruation.

Spasmodic dysmenorrhoea is common between the ages of 15 and 25 years, after which it usually, but not always, gradually resolves. It used to be relieved by dilatation of the cervix and it may be cured by a full-term pregnancy. On the other hand, the premenstrual syndrome may start at menarche and last until the menopause, with an increase in severity and incidence after the mid-30s, and an increase with parity.

Premenstrual syndrome increases at times of stress, while the severity of the pain in spasmodic dysmenorrhoea is unrelated to stress.

The sufferer of spasmodic dysmenorrhoea tends to be immature with small breasts, pink nipples, and scanty pubic and axillary hair. Premenstrual syndrome, however, may be found in all types of women, but usually the mature woman with large breasts. Table 19.1 summarises the difference between spasmodic dysmenorrhoea and premenstrual syndrome.

Lennane and Lennane (1973) have drawn attention to the fact that although spasmodic dysmenorrhoea has an obvious hormonal basis, being related to the presence of ovulation, it is too often alleged to be a psychogenic disorder. Premenstrual syndrome is likewise too often regarded as of psychogenic origin.

The importance of differentiating between spasmodic dysmenorrhoea and premenstrual syndrome lies in the response to treatment, for spasmodic dysmenorrhoea responds readily to prostaglandin inhibitors and to oestrogen, but premenstrual syndrome responds to progesterone. Even so, it is no longer necessary to resort to hormone therapy for spasmodic dysmenorrhoea unless the young woman also requires contraception.

The recent findings that sufferers of spasmodic dysmenorrhoea have a high level of prostaglandin F2α and E2 explains the benefit obtained from prostaglandin inhibitory drugs (Fuchs). Mefanamic acid, 250mg three times daily, is particularly effective against prostaglandin F2α, which not only removes the pain but also

Table 19.1

Differences between spasmodic dysmenorrhoea and premenstrual syndrome

	Spasmodic dysmenorrhoea	Premenstrual syndrome
Time of onset	Menstruation	Premenstruum
Site of pain	Uterine and ovarian nerve distribution	Lower abdomen, back, breasts, headaches, generalised joint pains
Type of pain	Spasmodic	Heavy, dragging, continuous
Age of onset	Two years after menarche	Menarche, pregnancy and pill
Predominant age group	15–25 years	Over 35 years
Effect of ovulation	Only present in ovular cycles	Present in ovular and anovular cycles
Premenstrual symptoms	Absent	Present
Effect of stress	Unrelated	Increased symptoms
Effect of pregnancy	Cures	Increases severity
Sexual development	Immature	Mature
Effect of pill	Cures	Increases symptoms
Treatment	Prostaglandin inhibitors, oestrogens or pill	Progesterone

decreases the amount of menstrual loss by 25%. Should the woman require contraception then the oestrogen-progestogen pill will remove the pain. Alternatively, if she does not obtain enough relief from prostaglandin inhibitors she may be given ethinyloestradiol in an initial dose of 50mg daily from days 5 to 25, with decreasing doses in subsequent months when full relief has been obtained. It is wise to continue for 6–9 months before trying a cycle without medication.

Endometriosis with its triad of dysmenorrhoea, infertility and dyspareunia may present with premenstrual symptoms. However, the correct diagnosis may be suspected on vaginal examination and confirmed by laparoscopy. While awaiting investigation such patients may usefully be started on pro-gestogens – for example norethisterone 10–30mg daily given continuously for several months – or with an anti-gonadotropin – for example, danazol 100–200mg three times daily.

20

Premenstrual syndrome and pre-eclampsia

During a survey into the incidence of premenstrual syndrome, 192 women were interviewed personally. All had suffered from pre-eclampsia during the previous eight years. The record card of the pre-eclamptic pregnancy was available and the interview started by reminding the woman that during the relevant pregnancy she had been ill for two weeks (or however long her records showed). The most frequent reaction was, 'No – the doctor said I was ill for two weeks, but in fact I was feeling ill throughout that pregnancy, and it was only the last two weeks that he agreed I was ill and he advised me to rest'. Many of these women experienced a normal pregnancy, after the affected one, and would compare their sense of well-being in a normal pregnancy with the experience of unremitting pregnancy symptoms during the pre-eclamptic one. Confirmatory evidence was in fact on most of the record cards, which had noted symptoms during the mid-trimester while blood pressure and weight gain were normal and no oedema or proteinuria were observed. Some cards bore such remarks as 'headaches referred to optician' or 'daily vomiting – given dietary advice'. The early days of pregnancy are usually accompanied by morning sickness and this is considered a natural discomfort of pregnancy, so that when the patient later mentions headache, vomiting, lethargy, irritability and depression, there is a natural tendency to assume that they are of a similar nature and therefore of little importance. Among these 192 mothers interviewed, 86% subsequently developed the premenstrual syndrome, and it was noted that the symptoms each woman had experienced during her pre-eclamptic pregnancy were the same as her present premenstrual symptoms. Figure 5.2 shows the symptoms the women experienced during their pre-eclamptic pregnancy and in the premenstruum (Dalton, 1954).

A prospective survey into the incidence of pregnancy symptoms was then undertaken at University College Hospital, London, where 633 antenatal patients were asked on only one occasion, between the 16th and 28th weeks of pregnancy, 'Do you feel as well now as you did before pregnancy started?' Those who gave a negative reply were further asked about their symptoms. Their subsequent history showed that among those who were feeling well at the time of the interview only 10% developed pre-eclampsia compared with 25% for those who had symptoms in the middle trimester. Figure 20.1 shows that those with symptoms had a higher incidence of severe pre-eclampsia, proteinuria, stillbirths and twins.

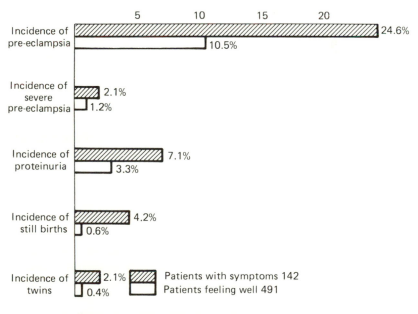

Fig. 20.1   Differences between patients with symptoms and those feeling well between 16th and 28th week of pregnancy. (From Dalton K. (1962). *J. Obs. Gynaec.*; Brit. Commonwealth. **69**:3.)

The type of pregnancy symptoms complained of are shown in Table 20.1.

Table 20.1

Pregnancy symptoms in the middle trimester in women who developed pre-eclampsia

Lethargy	88%
Nausea and vomiting	65%
Depression	52%
Paraesthesia	46%
Backache	44%
Headache	35%
Vertigo	26%
Fainting	12%

The similarity of premenstrual syndrome with pre-eclampsia was first noted in 1940 by Greenhill and Freed who suggested the title 'toxaemia of menstruation' as a companion to 'toxaemia of pregnancy'. As medical knowledge of the two diseases accumulates, the similarity becomes more marked. Both diseases have a first stage of symptoms, either premenstrual or pregnancy, which includes depression, irritability, lethargy, headache, backache, nausea and vertigo. These are present from mid-cycle or mid-pregnancy, and increase in severity as the cycle or pregnancy proceeds. This is followed by a stage of signs of oedema, weight gain, rise in blood pressure, and proteinuria which may also occur in premenstrual syndrome (Figs. 7.9, 7.10 and 7.11). These symptoms may ease with bed rest, whether in the premenstruum or pregnancy. Finally, if the disease progresses there is a stage of fits, either epileptic or eclamptic, both usually being preceded by a severe headache as a warning of the imminence of a fit (Table 20.2).

In view of the similarities, and the fact that premenstrual syndrome responds to progesterone if it is administered in the stage of symptoms and before the development of the stage of signs, progesterone has been used to relieve pregnancy symptoms in the middle trimester onwards until delivery (Dalton, 1957).

Figure 20.2 shows the effect of giving progesterone at the 24th week to a patient with pregnancy symptoms who was showing an excessive weight gain. Initially progesterone caused a weight loss

Table 20.2

Similarity of premenstrual syndrome and pre-eclampsia

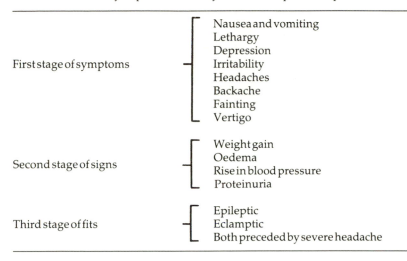

First stage of symptoms	Nausea and vomiting Lethargy Depression Irritability Headaches Backache Fainting Vertigo
Second stage of signs	Weight gain Oedema Rise in blood pressure Proteinuria
Third stage of fits	Epileptic Eclamptic Both preceded by severe headache

and then she had a normal pregnancy weight gain until she had a normal delivery at term (Dalton, 1955).

Progesterone trials in the prophylaxis of pre-eclampsia

Controlled trials were undertaken at Chase Farm Hospital, Enfield, where women presenting with pregnancy symptoms during the middle trimester were selected at random for inclusion in the symptomatic or progesterone-treated group. In these trials the incidence of pre-eclampsia was reduced from 11% in 66 controls to 3% among 62 progesterone-treated women (Dalton, 1962).

These controlled trials were later repeated at the City of London Maternity Hospital using the same protocol with similar random selection during the middle trimester, but using progesterone suppositories or pessaries instead of injections. The results of treatment with 400mg progesterone suppositories or pessaries daily or thrice daily succeeded in reducing the incidence of pre-eclampsia again from 11% in 88 controls to 3% in 80 progesterone-treated women (see Table 14.2).

Progesterone treatment

Women attending for antenatal examination should be asked

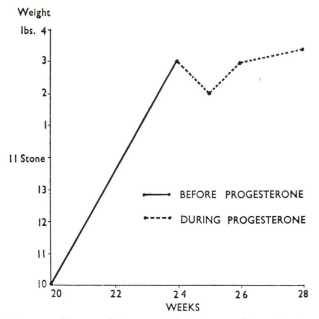

Primipara, 28 years. Oedema and heartburn at 24 weeks. Symptoms relieved by 100 mg i.m. progesterone. Maintained on 50 mg on alternate days from 24th week until normal delivery at term.

Fig. 20.2   The effect of progesterone on weight gain in pregnancy.

if they feel as well as they did before the pregnancy started, and any symptoms present should be noted on their antenatal records. Women complaining of lethargy, nausea and vomiting, depression, paraesthesia, backache, headache, vertigo or fainting should be given the option of receiving progesterone if two or more of these symptoms are present. Treatment should be started with progesterone suppositories or pessaries 400mg twice a day or intramuscular injections of 100mg daily for one week. If, when the woman returns, there has been symptomatic relief the dose should be continued for four weeks, and then if still free from symptoms the dose may be halved and then discontinued. On the other hand, if there has been no relief of symptoms the dose should be increased, using suppositories up to four times daily, or 200mg by intramuscular injections. Progesterone should be continued for as long as symptoms persist, if necessary until delivery.

Progesterone was isolated in 1932 (Allen) and only five years later there were reports of clinical trials into the use of progesterone in severe pre-eclampsia; at that time only 5mg were injected daily for four days (Marsden, Young, Paterson, McMann & Bennett). With their development in the 1950s progestogens were tried for the treatment of pre-eclampsia, until their use was abruptly halted with the realisation that in early pregnancy progestogens could cause masculinisation of the female fetus. Unfortunately, very few doctors understood the important differences between progestogens and progesterone (Oakley) so progesterone treatment of pre-eclampsia was stopped and has hardly been reconsidered since then. There have, however, been no reports of masculinisation following progesterone treatment (Dalton, 1981), but instead there has been the encouraging finding of enhanced intelligence and educational attainments in children whose mothers benefited from progesterone (Chapter 12) (Dalton, 1968 & 1976).

In 1975 Sammour and his colleagues in Egypt used injections of 50mg progesterone four times daily in 50 women. Ten were normal pregnant women and 40 were women with pre-eclampsia. In all cases the hypertension eased and there was a marked increase in the 24-hour urinary output with a loss of weight. Serum uric acid showed a significant drop and the urea clearance values also improved. The serum sodium showed a decline while the serum potassium did not show any marked variation.

Today we know that progesterone has an immunosuppressive property (Rothchild). This function would explain the 30-fold increase in the progesterone level during pregnancy which is needed to protect the fetus from the immunologically hostile environment of the mother. Today, pre-eclampsia is recognised as an autoimmune disease. The need to reinvestigate the place of progesterone in the prophylaxis of pre-eclampsia remains paramount. There is every possibility that the last chapter of the progesterone story in relation to pre-eclampsia is about to be written.

21

Premenstrual syndrome and postnatal depression

Marce, the French physician, was the first to point out in 1855 that as puerperal psychosis improved, the improvement occurred during the postmenstruum with a deterioration after ovulation until menstruation. This observation has been confirmed over the years (Boyd).

Schmidt in 1943 described such a case in a 21-year-old woman who was admitted to hospital with psychosis for five weeks, but: 'Two weeks after her return home she again developed the psychosis. On the fifth day she began menstruating, and the psychosis cleared up one week after the period. For two weeks she was apparently normal, attending her household duties and going about as usual. At the end of two weeks the psychosis returned. She again menstruated on the fifth day and the psychosis terminated one week after the menstrual period. On the third month the psychosis advanced five days and suddenly disappeared with the advent of menstruation. The onset of the psychosis could be noted several days in advance by slight irritability; otherwise the patient was apparently normal during the sane phases.'

Recognising the hormonal relationship Schmidt treated her with 1mg progesterone injections for three days from ovulation and then increased to 10mg progesterone daily: '. . . with immediate effect on the symptoms. The nervousness and irritability disappeared; the patient became more calm and so continued with daily injections. In spite of the dread of the hypodermics the patient readily admitted that the injections had a most soothing effect. The cumulative action of the hormone was very apparent. There was practically a minor change of personality. The patient became more congenial and developed an intense interest in both her household duties and other diversions. Her mental acumen was far superior to that noted in any of the normal phases since the onset of psychosis. There was no indication of recurrence.'

The gradual transition of postnatal depression to premenstrual syndrome is shown in Fig. 21.1. In stage one the severity of the symptoms continues unabated day by day, then there is stage two in which the symptoms increase before and ease after menstruation. Finally, there is stage three in which the symptoms are absent in the postmenstruum but return each premenstruum, thus conforming to the definition of premenstrual syndrome (Dalton, 1980). The high incidence of premenstrual syndrome following postnatal depression was also noted by Malleson & Hegarty.

Types

Postnatal depression must be seen as a spectrum with the severity of symptoms ranging from normality through maternity blues and postnatal depression to psychosis, with the entities imperceptibly merging one into another (Fig. 21.2).

Maternity blues was described by Pitt (1973) as a mother having tears or feeling temporarily depressed during the first ten days postpartum and was present in half the 100 women he studied. He concluded that it is 'such a trivial, fleeting commonplace disorder that the pregnant mother should be warned to expect it to avoid being taken by surprise'. The episodes of crying usually last no more than five minutes, but they may cry continuously for two hours or more. The crying is not necessarily resulting from sadness, but for a variety of reasons such as when they see the birth announcement or receive a bouquet of roses. They are oversensitive to rebuffs (Yalom *et al.*).

Postnatal depression occurs in some 7–10% of women, in whom the blues does not disappear within two weeks but gradually increases with depression developing (Ryle, Tod, Pitt & Dalton, 1971). As with premenstrual depression, postnatal depression has all the usual characteristics of an endogenous depression but with the added symptoms of irritability, irrationality and impatience, with a weight gain instead of loss, food craving

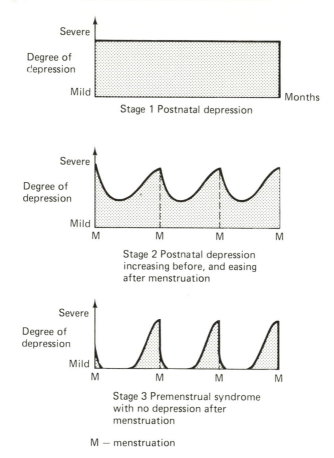

Fig. 21.1   Stages as postnatal depression changes to premenstrual syndrome. (From Dalton K. (1980). *Depression After Childbirth,* Oxford University Press.)

instead of anorexia and a yearning for sleep, which is constantly interrupted by baby crying at night. The onset may occur immediately after birth, on starting oral contraceptives, on stopping lactation or with the onset of the first menstruation. These patients need medical attention for there is the ever-present possibility that they may injure themselves, their babies or their husbands.

Puerperal psychosis occurs in one in 200 to 500 cases after child-birth. The patient is obviously mentally ill with confusion,

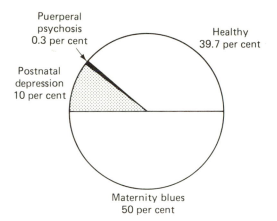

Fig. 21.2 Frequency of postnatal illnesses. (From Dalton K. (1980). *Depression After Childbirth,* Oxford University Press.)

delusions, mania or hallucinations and is at risk of hurting herself or her baby; she requires urgent hospital admission.

Characteristics of postnatal depression

A prospective study was carried out in 1971 of postnatal depression treated by a group of 14 general practitioners and a psychiatrist centred on the North Middlesex Hospital, London, a general district hospital (Dalton, 1971). The characteristics noted were as follows:

1. Favourable attitude to motherhood, as shown by welcoming the pregnancy, being elated during pregnancy and free from pregnancy symptoms, enthusiastic about and successful at lactation.
2. Labile emotions, anxious at the time of the first interview, elated during pregnancy, and depressed during the puerperium.

Risk of recurrence

To study the risk of recurrence in those who had previously suffered from postnatal depression severe enough to require medical treatment, a survey was carried out of 413 women attending for treatment of premenstrual syndrome, who also had a history of postnatal depression. These women had a total of 915 full-term pregnancies; 88 women had only one pregnancy (many had been advised to have no further pregnancies because of the risk of a return of postnatal depression). There were a further 104 women with more than one child, but who had no further pregnancy after the one affected by postnatal depression. Of the 221 women who had a subsequent pregnancy after the one complicated by postnatal depression there was a recurrence rate of 68%, increasing among those whose illness had required hospital admission to 84% (Fig. 21.3) (Dalton, 1980).

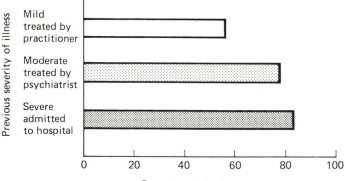

Fig. 21.3   Risk of recurrence of postnatal depression in subsequent pregnancy (221 pregnancies). (From Dalton K. (1980). *Depression After Childbirth,* Oxford University Press.)

The recurrence rate was not 100% however, and there appeared to be no way of predicting who or which pregnancy would be followed by postnatal depression. The survey included five women who all had six pregnancies with at least one which was complicated by postnatal depression, but the order of the postnatal depression varied in each case (Fig. 21.4).

The 413 women studied had experienced a total of 915 full-term pregnancies, of which 609 had been complicated by post-natal depression. Table 21.1 shows the incidence of obstetric complications during a normal puerperium and one complicated by postnatal depression, with no difference noted in respect of pre-eclampsia, stillbirths or neonatal deaths, abnormality in the baby or twins. There was a higher incidence of threatened abortions but these did not reach a level of statistical significance. The average age of women developing postnatal depression was

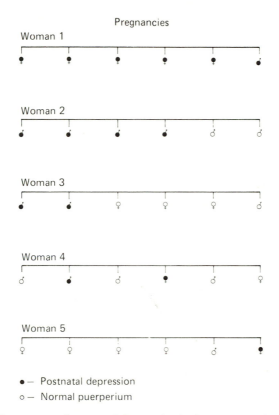

Fig. 21.4   Occurrence of postnatal depression in five women who each had six pregnancies. (From Dalton K. (1980). *Depression After Childbirth.* Oxford University Press.)

25.4 years in those requiring hospital admission and 26.2 years among women with mild postnatal depression treated by their general practitioner.

Incidence

Postnatal depression is no more frequent among those who have had a previous psychiatric history or who had a complicated pregnancy delivery; suffered a stillbirth or neonatal death; nor does it appear related to religion (Founder *et al.*), cultural differences, or to civilisation (Dalton, 1980). It can occur after a spontaneous or therapeutic abortion. As with premenstrual syndrome there does appear to be a genetic factor, several women

Table 21.1

Incidence of obstetric complications in normal puerperium
and in postnatal depression

n	Normal puerperium 306	Postnatal depression 609	Total 915
Pre-eclampsia	27 (8.8%)	58 (9.5%)	85
Stillbirth/neonatal death	3 (1.0%)	5 (0.8%)	8
Abnormality in baby	4 (1.3%)	12 (2.0%)	16
Twins	5 (1.6%)	6 (1.0%)	11
Threatened abortion	6 (2.0%)	30 (4.9%)	36

reporting that their mothers were admitted to hospital with psychosis following their birth, and if one identical twin suffers the other is likely to suffer similarly.

In the 100 consecutive hospital cases of severe premenstrual syndrome there had been 59 pregnancies (including six abortions) in which puerperal depression, sufficient to need psychiatric or medical care, had occurred in 73%. Viewed from another angle, if a patient has puerperal depression, the chance of premenstrual syndrome subsequently developing is almost 90%.

Postnatal depression followed by premenstrual syndrome

When taking case histories from mothers with premenstrual syndrome it is remarkable how frequently the onset of their premenstrual syndrome follows on from a pregnancy complicated by puerperal depression. One hears such expressions as 'I've never been the same since my child was born' or, 'I haven't got over my last pregnancy', which may have been up to ten years previously.

A factory worker with severe depression stated that the onset of her illness had occurred four years previously. Later the husband was interviewed; he referred to the seven years of his wife's illness. She had two children, aged seven and four years, and on both occasions she had received antidepressant drugs during the year following each birth, and premenstrual depression had continued ever since, increasing in severity after the second postnatal depression.

This is confirmed by the high incidence of postnatal depression,

58% being noted in women with premenstrual syndrome when interviewed at their first consultation (Tables 8.3, 27.11).

Prophylactic treatment

During pregnancy the progesterone level rises gradually over the months of pregnancy to a level some 30 to 50 times the peak level reached in the mid-luteal phase (Hoffmann & v Làm), and then at delivery there is a sudden abrupt fall in progesterone from about 150ng/ml at the end of the pregnancy to a mere 7ng/ml on the third day after birth and thereafter it is barely discernible in the blood (Fig. 12.1). Postnatal depression is thought to be due to a failure of adaptation to the precipitous drop in the progesterone level. Progesterone prophylactic therapy is therefore aimed at easing this abrupt drop by giving progesterone supplement during the puerperium and until menstruation is re-established. After completion of delivery the patient is given 100mg progesterone intramuscularly daily for seven days followed by progesterone suppositories or pessaries 400mg twice daily for the next two months or the return of menstruation, with permission for the patient to increase the dose of suppositories or pessaries up to six daily if necessary. It has been successfully used by the author for the last 20 years. Soltau and Taylor also reported its successful use (1982).

Prophylactic progesterone trials

The author's survey of prophylactic progesterone in the last three years is described in the following paragraphs.

For the purpose of the survey postnatal depression was defined as the first psychiatric illness in a woman with no previous psychiatric illness, which occurred within six months of delivery and was severe enough to require medical help. Pregnant women who have previously required treatment for postnatal depression were offered prophylactic progesterone and, if they agreed, letters of instruction were sent to their general practitioners and their obstetricians. They were both asked to arrange for these women to receive 100mg progesterone intramuscularly on completion of labour and daily for the next seven days, followed by suppositories or pessaries 400mg twice daily for two months or until menstruation returned. The women were instructed to obtain their progesterone supplies in late pregnancy to avoid any difficulty when arriving at hospital for delivery. They were followed up by interview or written report at six months. Thirty-three women accepted progesterone prophylaxis, but in two cases the obstetrician would not agree. The 31 treated women had previously had a total of 66 pregnancies. They had experienced 46 full-time pregnancies of which 42 (91%) had been followed by postnatal depression, 13 spontaneous abortions followed by four cases of postnatal depression and seven therapeutic abortions followed by three postnatal depressions. Their previous episodes of postnatal depression had been classified as 'mild' requiring treatment by a general practitioner in 27 cases, 'moderate' requiring treatment by a consultant psychiatrist in eight cases, and 'severe' requiring hospital admissions in 14 cases. Nine women received electroconvulsive treatment.

All these 31 women who had received progesterone prophylaxis were delivered of healthy babies (14 boys and 17 girls).

One woman had pre-eclampsia requiring antenatal admission, one was depressed in pregnancy, one delivery was by repeat Caesarean section, one woman had postpartum haemorrhage at two weeks, when she was advised to stop progesterone treatment. Twenty-four were still breastfeeding at three months. Two women developed postnatal depression. One woman, who was advised to stop progesterone after her curettage at two weeks, relapsed within a few days of stopping progesterone and required admission to hospital. Another woman had an acute psychotic episode at eight months postnatally on stopping lactation and starting menstruation. Her attack responded within three days of restarting progesterone injections and she had no further relapse. Two other mothers had traumatic experiences. One had a cot death at two weeks and another found her husband in bed with another woman four weeks postnatally: neither developed postnatal depression. One of the two women whose obstetrician was unwilling to cooperate developed postnatal depression.

Thus these 31 women had an incidence of 6% postnatal depression compared with their previous incidence of 91% after full-term pregnancies, or the expected recurrence rate of 68% (Fig. 21.5). Progesterone prophylactic treatment is simple and harmless, it enhances lactation and there appear to be no side effects.

The results of prophylactic progesterone in another group of women seen during 1982 is shown in Table 27.32.

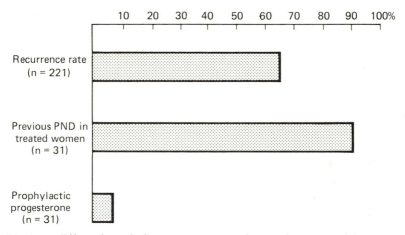

Fig. 21.5   Effect of prophylactic progesterone therapy for postnatal depression (PND).

Treatment of established postnatal depression

As stated in Chapter 12 progesterone treatment is essentially prophylactic; when postnatal depression has developed, progesterone will only prevent the exacerbation that may be expected in the premenstruum. It is necessary to continue other antidepressive or antipsychotic medication while the illness is in stages 1 and 2. Once improvement has occurred and the postnatal depression changed to premenstrual syndrome then the other medication may be gradually reduced and then stopped but the progesterone treatment should be continued as long as it is required.

One looks ahead to the day when prophylactic progesterone therapy will be routine, and postnatal depression a rarity.

22

The outcome of pregnancy

Pregnancy disturbs the normal rhythm of premenstrual syndrome. At the time of the first missed menstruation the usual premenstrual symptoms become more severe and prolonged until they gradually merge into the symptoms of pregnancy, especially morning sickness, tiredness and tenderness and enlargement of the breasts. Patients who are receiving progesterone for the relief of premenstrual symptoms are advised to continue with the progesterone treatment until the pregnancy is confirmed. If symptoms have resolved, the treatment can then be stopped.

After the first trimester most sufferers from premenstrual syndrome are free from their usual symptoms of asthma, migraine, epilepsy and depression and enjoy their pregnancy. In a small minority, however, the symptoms persist and treatment will need to be continued to full term. It is among this latter group that the candidates for pre-eclampsia will be found (Chapter 20).

Defective luteal phase
A defective luteal phase is now recognised as a cause of infertility in some normal ovulating women. It may be recognised by an indecisive, stepwise rise in the basal body temperature after ovulation, by a luteal phase lasting 12 days or less, by a timed endometrial biopsy or serial progesterone assays. The luteal phase may be prolonged, enabling a pregnancy to be achieved, by progesterone administration starting two to four days after ovulation and continued until pregnancy is confirmed (Jones).

The recommended dose is 50–400mg by suppository or pessary, or 25–100mg daily injections. It might be mentioned that progesterone suppositories 50mg for the correction of defective luteal phase are considered safe and efficacious by the American Federal Drug Administration (see also Appendix Table 27.30).

Hyperemesis

In patients who are suffering from hyperemesis gravidarum or severe pregnancy symptoms (lethargy, irritability, depression, headache and nausea), relief may be obtained within two days by giving an injection of progesterone 100mg once or twice daily and continued until the symptoms are resolved. Then a maintenance dose is required of progesterone suppositories 400mg up to four times daily until the patient has been free from symptoms for about two weeks. By the 16th week the symptoms have usually subsided and by the 20th week the woman will begin to experience the feeling of wellbeing so often associated with a normal pregnancy, or she may even feel 'better than ever', free from any premenstrual symptoms and elated; this coincides with a high placental progesterone level.

Spontaneous abortions

There are probably as many different causes of fetal deaths as in any other age group. Nevertheless, there is one group of women who, having developed hyperemesis or increasingly severe pregnancy symptoms, abort spontaneously between the 8th and 14th week. Occasionally, after several weeks of daily vomiting the symptoms end abruptly and a day or two later the woman has a spontaneous abortion, the fetus having died when the symptoms stopped.

In these cases where a spontaneous abortion follows on an increasing hyperemesis, which ends with, or just before the fetal loss, it is suggested that deficiency of progesterone is an important factor and the patient should be offered prophylactic progesterone to remove pregnancy symptoms in her subsequent pregnancies.

Threatened abortion

Women who have threatened abortions may be divided into two groups, viz those with hyperemesis or pregnancy symptoms and those who have been free from pregnancy symptoms. In the first group of women it seems that relief of pregnancy symptoms with progesterone helps by raising the progesterone level until the placental output is adequate to maintain the pregnancy. Johansson found that the mean progesterone level at the ninth week of pregnancy was significantly lower than at the fifth week (Fig. 10.3) and suggested that the placenta does not replace the corpus luteum as a major source of progesterone until about the ninth week.

A series of 24 women who threatened to abort and had a positive pregnancy test were treated within 24 hours of the onset of bleeding with intensive progesterone therapy sufficient to bring relief of pregnancy symptoms (Table 22.1). There was a significant difference in the outcome of pregnancy among those 15 women with pregnancy symptoms of whom 10 (66%) had a normal delivery of a live healthy baby, compared with the nine women who had no pregnancy symptoms of whom only one (9%) had a normal delivery (P=<0.01).

Table 22.1

Progesterone treatment of threatened abortion

Outcome of pregnancy	Abortion	Normal delivery	Total
Pregnancy symptoms	5	10	15
No pregnancy symptoms	8	1	9

Probability=<0.01

Progesterone treatment for habitual abortion

Progesterone was used in patients with habitual abortion 25 years ago. Progesterone pellets 6×25mg were implanted during the first trimester. There were conflicting reports of the efficiency of this treatment. Bishop and his colleagues claimed 86% success in those with two previous abortions and 75% with four or more previous abortions. On the other hand, Swyer and Daley, in controlled trials, found no significant difference among the treated and control patients.

Progestogens, believed to be true progesterone substitutes, then became the vogue for treatment of habitual and threatened abortion, but with the realisation that progestogens produced masculinisation of the female fetus all treatment, with both progesterone and progestogens, was stopped. With our present knowledge it is obvious that the dose of progesterone was far too small and there was no differentiation between patients with increasing hyperemesis and pregnancy symptoms, and those who were free from symptoms. Clinical experience suggests that when patients, in whom increasingly severe hyperemesis or pregnancy symptoms have preceded an abortion, are treated with progesterone during their next pregnancy, it has helped maintain the pregnancy.

Ideally, the progesterone should be administered as soon as there are pregnancy symptoms and before there is any blood loss or threat to the fetus. Many pregnancies have been observed where women with a history of three or more spontaneous abortions, accompanied by hyperemesis or increasingly severe pregnancy symptoms, have been treated with progesterone and the pregnancy has gone on to full term. Among them were two women each of whom had nine previous spontaneous abortions; they were both treated with progesterone and delivered at full term in the City of London Maternity Hospital. The use of progesterone therapy in this selected group of habitual aborters needs further assessment.

Premature labour

Csapa and his colleagues noted that women who went into premature labour of unknown cause had a marked deficiency of progesterone and precociously increased uterine activity. They suggested progesterone treatment in such cases, adding the rider, 'Can progesterone levels be increased exogenously in the third trimester when the source of progesterone is interuterinal placenta and the progesterone transport to the uterus is local rather than systemic?'

It would seem that before the potential progesterone therapy can be fully appreciated there must be a change of attitude among those responsible for obstetric care. The expectant mother must be positively asked about pregnancy symptoms, and consideration should be given to these rather than total reliance on the presence of abnormal signs – for example, bleeding, weight gain, hypertension or proteinuria – which occur later in pregnancy.

Prognosis of premenstrual syndrome

Three types of menstruation are found in women: that which is symptom free; spasmodic dysmenorrhoea; and that which occurs with the premenstrual syndrome. During pregnancy, most of those women who have symptom-free menstruation or spasmodic dysmenorrhoea will tend to have normal pregnancies, but the occasional woman will develop pre-eclampsia. On the other hand, sufferers from the premenstrual syndrome will in the main be free from their usual symptoms during pregnancy and be 'better than ever', but one in ten will develop pre-eclampsia (Fig. 22.1) (Dalton).

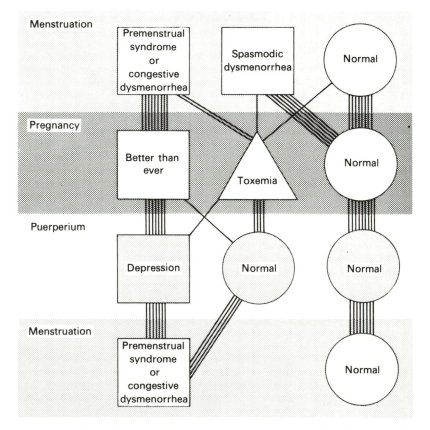

Fig. 22.1 Effect of pregnancy on menstruation. (From Dalton K. (1969). *The Menstrual Cycle*, Penguin Books.)

During the puerperium it will be those women who were elated and 'better than ever' in pregnancy who will be candidates for puerperal depression, while a woman who had a normal pregnancy or one complicated by pre-eclampsia may expect to feel normal during the puerperium.

When menstruation recurs after pregnancy 90% of those who have suffered from pre-eclampsia or postnatal depression can expect to suffer from premenstrual syndrome, whereas those who had a normal pregnancy may expect to have normal painfree menstruation (Fig. 22.1). However, if progesterone has been used for the prophylaxis of pre-eclampsia or postnatal depression the chances of premenstrual syndrome developing are diminished.

23

The menopause

Hormonal changes

With the disappearance of the ovarian follicles and the ovarian production of oestrogen at the menopause there is an interference with the normal feedback pathways. The hypothalamus and pituitary increase their production of releasing factors and gonadotrophins to stimulate the ovaries, which are no longer able to respond (Fig. 23.1). The gonadotrophin levels may show a tenfold increase at this time, and these levels remain raised for some 16–20 years after the menopause and then gradually decline, but still remain higher than the mean values during the menstruating years (Cooke).

The pronounced increase in the levels of FSH and LH and the decrease in oestradiol at the menopause make differential diagnosis easy by an estimation of these hormone levels. Thus amenorrhoea due to stress in a normal menstruating woman can readily be distinguished from amenorrhoea due to a premature menopause. Similarly, it is possible to recognise those whose ovaries are still functioning after a hysterectomy by their normal levels of oestrogen, FSH and LH.

Following bilateral oophorectomy there is an increase in plasma FSH levels after six to eight days and in the plasma LH levels after eight to ten days. Within three weeks there is a threefold increase in plasma FSH and a twofold increase in plasma LH (Lauritzen).

The main oestrogen excreted from the ovary is oestradiol, but after the menopause oestrone, a much weaker oestrogen, is synthesised in the fat, liver and other peripheral tissues from

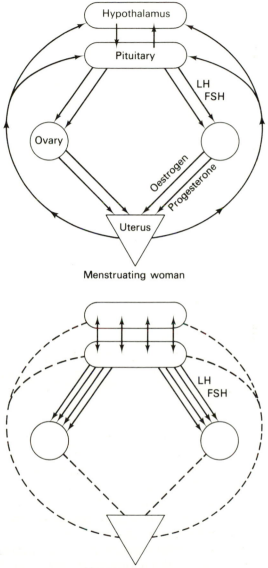

Fig. 23.1 Hormonal pathways in menstruating and menopausal women.

oestrogen precursors produced by the adrenals. There is no compensatory hypertrophy of the adrenals to help in this extra production of the oestrogen precursors. After the menopause, progesterone is no longer required for the proliferation of the endometrium and as progesterone has been synthesised in the adrenals during the menstruating years, there is usually enough to cope with the postmenopausal years. Thus premenstrual symptoms may be expected to end two years after the last menstruation. Of the many women with severe premenstrual syndrome who have been observed from their mid-40s through the menopause there have been two whose cyclical symptoms have continued until 67 years, but they must be considered rarities.

Premenopausal years

During the premenopausal years there is frequently an increase in the intensity of premenstrual syndrome, thus some women find that premenstrual symptoms which were once bearable and acceptable and requiring only mild analgesia have now become incapacitating and need medical attention. About 10% of women state their premenstrual syndrome started at the menopause, although far more women during their early 40s erroneously blame the menopause for their premenstrual symptoms (Greene & Dalton).

The last menstruation

In Britain the mean age of the last menstruation is 50 years, with a range from 45 to 55 years. In sufferers from premenstrual syndrome the last menstruation is likely to occur after 50 years, while those who initially suffered from spasmodic dysmenor-rhoea tend to end menstruation earlier. There is a marked family similarity in the time of the menopause. In some families all the female members end early, while in others they have a late ending. There may be a correlation between the age of menarche and that of the menopause, those starting the menarche early tend to have a late menopause. Another factor which appears to influence the age of the menopause is heavy smoking, which may advance the expected time by about one year.

Types of ending

There are three common types of ending to menstruation, although any combination may occur.

1. Gradual ending with decreasing loss (Fig. 23.2) (Dalton, 1969).
2. Missed menstruation with increasing irregularity (Fig. 23.3).
3. Abrupt ending (Fig. 23.4).

It is when there is an abrupt ending that pregnancy is feared, but vaginal examination will reveal either the warm, red, moist vagina with a soft cervix characteristic of pregnancy, or pale, dry vagina with firm cervix suggestive of the menopause. The abrupt ending is also more frequently associated with depression. Often there is a possibility of the 'empty-nest syndrome', with the history of one or more children leaving home for employment, college or marriage. Charting the days of the depression, however, may confirm its presence during the premenstruum followed by freedom from symptoms during the postmenstruum, or may disclose the presence of cyclical menopausal depression, which differentiates it from the empty-nest syndrome.

Cyclical menopausal syndrome

For most sufferers the menopause marks the end of their pre-menstrual syndrome; however, there is a minority in whom cyclical symptoms continue after the menopause.

A 55-year-old married housewife with two children experienced a gradual onset of periodic depression coinciding with the cessation of menstruation at the age of 47 years. She received antidepressant drug therapy for the first two years from her general practitioner, and then was admitted to a psychiatric hospital when she developed suicidal ideas. Psychotherapy and drug therapy were of no avail, and electroconvulsive therapy brought only temporary relief, so finally at the age of 54 years she underwent a cortical undercut leucotomy. When first seen she was still severly incapacitated by her periodical depressions. The onset of an attack was preceded by a day of agitation and swelling of the face and fingers. She would then go to bed and lie staring at the ceiling all day, too apathetic to move. The attacks

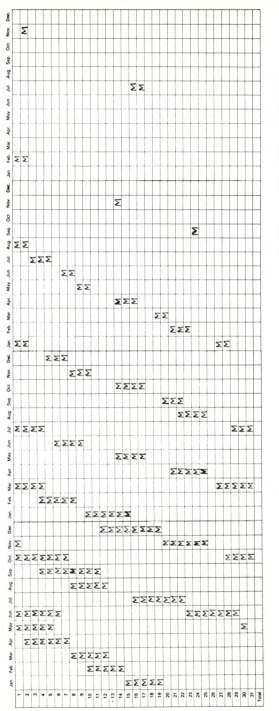

Fig. 23.2 Gradual ending of menstruation. (From Dalton K. (1969). *The Menstrual Cycle*, Penguin Books.)

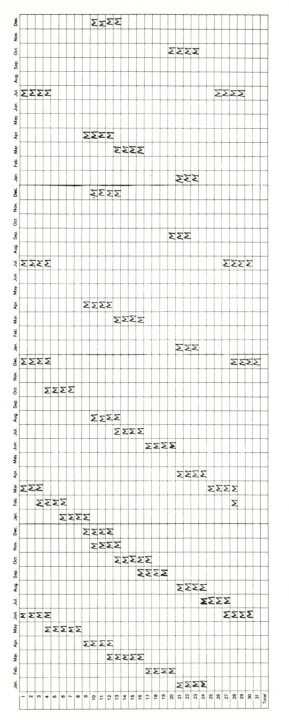

Fig. 23.3   Increasing irregularity of menstruation. (From Dalton K. (1969). *The Menstrual Cycle*, Penguin Books.)

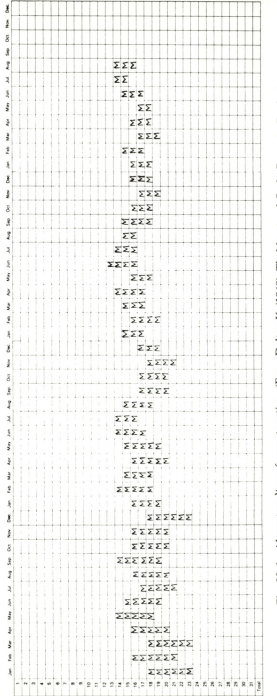

Fig. 23.4 Abrupt ending of menstruation. (From Dalton K. (1969). *The Menstrual Cycle*, Penguin Books.)

would last from 7 to 14 days. During her two pregnancies she had felt exceedingly well, but they had been followed by short-lived attacks of postnatal depression. The monthly rhythm of attacks was first noticed by the husband, who stated that they were similar to, but of longer duration than, attacks of depression she had suffered with her menstruation in the early days of married life. The husband was advised to record the days his wife spent in bed. The record of her depressed days suggested monthly cyclical attacks (Fig. 23.5); and she was treated with progesterone in gradually increasing doses. She became completely free from symptoms and was leading an active social life on treatment with progesterone injections 100mg daily. After two years it was possible to stop treatment without a recurrence of symptoms (Dalton, 1964).

Alcoholic excess is also frequent at the menopause, and careful observation of women may differentiate those whose drinking bouts occur only in association with scanty menstrual bleeding or at the time of the missed menstruation. This is a worthwhile differentiation, for those women with cyclical alcoholic excess can receive positive therapeutic help from progesterone for an otherwise difficult and often hopeless condition. Tragically, one husband handed in a chart, after his wife had died from an alcoholic debauch, showing seven months of cyclical attacks of alcoholism.

The increase in shoplifting in women in their fourth and fifth decades has been attributed to the cyclical depression and absentmindedness of women with this syndrome.

The commonest physical symptoms are vertigo, syncope, and rheumatic pains of the joints and muscles, the latter especially so among the obese. Water retention and obesity are common at this time.

The effect of an artificial menopause

Women who have suffered discomfort and crippling symptoms during the paramenstruum will naturally look forward to the time when these sufferings will end. Those who are advised to have an hysterectomy and/or oophorectomy know this means the end of menstruation and hope it will also relieve the attendant symptoms. Sufferers from spasmodic dysmenorrhoea and endo-metriosis can certainly expect relief of pain after a hysterectomy,

	Jan.	Feb.	Mar.	Apr.	May	Jun.	Jul.	Aug.	Sep.	Oct.	Nov.	Dec.
1									X			
2									X			
3									X			
4									X			
5								X	X			
6								X	X			
7							X	X	X	X		
8							X	X	X	X		
9							X	X	X	X		
10							X	X	X	X	X	
11							X	X	X	X	X	
12							X	X	X	X	X	
13							X			X	X	
14							X			X	X	
15							X			X	X	
16							X			X	X	
17							X			X	X	
18										X		
19										X		
20										X		
21										X		
22										X		
23										X		
24										X		
25										X		
26												
27												
28												
29												
30												
31							X					
Total												

Married Housewife, 55 years, Para 2.
X = days spent in bed, apathetic and depressed.

Fig. 23.5 Cyclical depression eight years after ending menstruation.

but sufferers from premenstrual syndrome should be warned that they are unlikely to be relieved of their recurrent premenstrual symptoms by the operation; indeed, they may well increase in severity. Dennerstein and Ryan (1982) in their review of medical publications emphasise the high incidence of psychological and sexual sequelae following hysterectomy, and this is particularly marked among those with preoperative psychological problems; this also includes women with premenstrual syndrome. The menstrual controlling centre in the brain is traumatised by a hysterectomy, but will usually settle down in 6–12 months and thereafter the cyclical symptoms will return. One surgeon who is known to diagnose premenstrual syndrome in his patients tells them it is due to a deficiency of progesterone, performs a hysterectomy and then refers them to the clinic for progesterone replacement therapy.

Cyclical symptoms after hysterectomy

There is frequently an interval of 6–12 months after a hysterectomy before cyclical symptoms recur, and these may be quite mild at the onset but gradually increase in severity over the next few months. Hence, the cyclical nature of recurrent symptoms may not be obvious for a year or two.

The diagnosis of recurrent cyclical symptoms in women who have previously had artificial menopause depends entirely on the charting of their symptoms. It is interesting that when a patient returns with a two to three month record of symptoms, it is often possible to remind her of the previous length of her cycle, for a short or long cycle is readily distinguishable. The duration of the symptoms also reflects the length of previous premenstrual attacks, either drawn out and lasting for 10–14 days, or an acute severe one of only one or two days' duration (Fig. 23.6) (Dalton, 1957).

Other patients who have had symptom-free menstruation may find that after a hysterectomy cyclical symptoms appear for the first time, as in the following patient.

At the age of 38 a single woman working as a housekeeper had a hysterectomy for menorrhagia due to fibroids. After the operation she was never really well and lost 19kg. She suffered from numerous headaches and complained of lethargy and depression. Two years later she received psychiatric treatment, which continued over the next eight years both as an inpatient and as an outpatient and included drug therapy and psychotherapy. When 48 years old she was referred by the psychiatrist for 'chronic anxiety and phobic symptoms which dated from hysterectomy'. At the interview the patient described how her attacks of depression were usually self-limiting, lasting 4–8 days, and

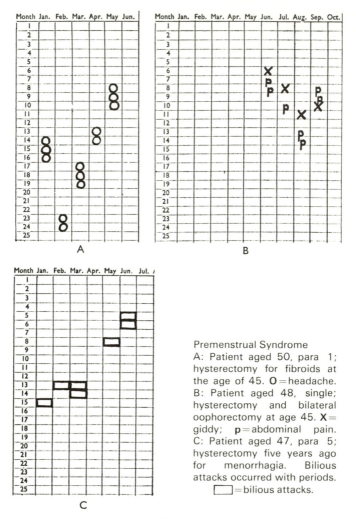

Premenstrual Syndrome
A: Patient aged 50, para 1; hysterectomy for fibroids at the age of 45. O = headache.
B: Patient aged 48, single; hysterectomy and bilateral oophorectomy at age 45. X = giddy; p = abdominal pain.
C: Patient aged 47, para 5; hysterectomy five years ago for menorrhagia. Bilious attacks occurred with periods. ☐ = bilious attacks.

Fig. 23.6 Cyclical symptoms after hysterectomy and oophorectomy.

accompanied by panic states, headaches and vertigo. Her chart showed the familiar patterns of symptoms in cycles of 28–33 days. After her first month's treatment with progesterone the patient reported a gradual improvement, 'feeling feminine again, working well, placid'. Four months later she was completely free from symptoms, happy and anxious to tackle again her previous employment as warden of a hostel for businesswomen, a task which called for considerable responsibility, a pleasant manner and even temper (Dalton, 1964).

The periodic attacks of lethargy, irritability and depression among sufferers make them feel difficult to live with, as shown by the fact that 44% of the married women in one series of post-hysterectomy women had either divorced, separated or sought the assistance of a marriage guidance counsellor since the operation (Dalton, 1957). While attacks of tension are related to menstruation the husband may be sympathetic to his marital partner, knowing that such an attack will soon end and feeling that it has an organic basis. However, after the operation the unaccountable and unexpected attacks of irritability strain the domestic harmony. As one husband put it, 'She used to have a reason for it, but now she's quite unpredictable', or another, 'I hoped the operation would make her more even-tempered'. Indeed, one remarked, 'Since the hysteria operation my wife's been more hysterical than ever'.

One woman wrote imploring for help stating 'I had a hysterectomy two years ago, the pattern of premenstrual tension reasserted itself so that there are, as in the past, only about ten days in the month when I feel optimistic and cheerful. Since then my marriage has begun to break up and I would like at the very least to eliminate the cause of friction.'

One survey of cyclical symptoms occurring after a hysterectomy (Dalton, 1957) showed the following:

Headaches	74%
Depression	62%
Vertigo	60%
Lethargy	57%
Joint and muscle pains	50%

Patients who develop symptoms after an artificial menopause are amenable to treatment. Keeping regular charts of symptoms after the operation is important for the differentiation between those whose symptoms are cyclical, and therefore likely to respond to the cyclical hormone progesterone, and those whose symptoms are continuous and likely to respond best to oestrogens. Explanation of the cyclical nature of their symptoms, and the knowledge that such symptoms are likely to continue until the time of the natural menopause, helps many women to accept symptoms. Where possible it is helpful to explain to the husband that his wife will still tend to have her monthly attacks of irritability and her 'off days' after a hysterectomy, until the expected time of her natural menopause. (See Appendix and Tables 27.24 to 27.29.)

Hormonal studies

The persistence of cyclical symptoms after a hysterectomy in women who previously suffered from premenstrual syndrome has been demonstrated by Bäckström and his colleagues (1981). They selected seven women preoperatively who had been advised a hysterectomy for fibromyoma or for menorrhagia and who suffered from tension, irritability and depression during the seven to ten premenstrual days, with a substantial decrease in symptoms within three days of starting menstruation and absence of symptoms in the postmentruum. Hormonal studies were carried out preoperatively and the women were admitted during their luteal phase. At operation, in addition to the hysterectomy the corpus luteum was enucleated, with the patient's permission, thus terminating prematurely the luteal phase to ensure that the patient could not know when the next menstruation should have started. Hormone studies continued for at least two months postoperatively, and the ovarian function persisted as indicated by the changes in the excretion of pregnanediol and total oestrogen. Cyclical changes in mood persisted after hysterectomy, with the greatest mental and physical symptoms occurring during the later luteal phase of the cycle. They concluded that neither the presence of the uterus nor the occurrence of menstruation are necessary for the manifestation of premenstrual syndrome, and this is further evidence that premenstrual syndrome has a hormonal basis.

Depression after hysterectomy

While surveys show a high incidence of depression after hysterectomy it is not known what proportion has a cyclical depression or a continuous depression (Barker & Richards). The cyclical depression is likely to be hormonal in origin, whereas the continuous depression may be of psychological aetiology. One might suspect that many would have responded to hormone therapy with either progesterone or oestrogen. Posthysterectomy depression is most likely to occur in the following patients:

1. Under 40 years of age at the time of the operation.
2. Previous history of depression, especially postnatal depression.
3. No gynaecological abnormality detected at operation. (In one of the surveys 45% of the uteri were reported to be normal.)
4. History of marital disruption.
5. Previous sterilisation.

Treatment of cyclical symptoms

Treatment of patients with cyclical symptoms which recur at the time of missed menstruation, following either a natural or artificial menopause, respond well to continuous progesterone. This can be administered initially by the rectal or vaginal route, and if the patient becomes free from symptoms she can have a progesterone implant, which in these circumstances usually lasts about 12 months.

Oestrogen deficiency symptoms

The specific symptoms of oestrogen deficiency are as follows:

1. Hot flushes, either visible or invisible, and drenching night sweats.
2. Atrophy of the vaginal epithelium, which in turn leads to pruritus and local soreness, dyspareunia and loss of libido, dysuria and frequency often diagnosed as 'cystitis'.
3. Osteoarthrosis and osteoporosis which present as generalised fleeting joint pains, especially of the feet and hands with stiffness on rising in the morning. If osteoporosis is pronounced there is a rise in urinary and blood calcium and in alkaline phosphatase, and later an increased incidence of fractures, especially of the wrists, neck of the femur and crushed vertebrae.

Non-specific symptoms which may occur at this time and may respond to oestrogen include headaches, depression, lethargy, forgetfulness, absent-mindedness, anxiety and loss of memory.

Diagnosis of oestrogen deficiency

Blood hormonal estimations are invaluable for the diagnosis of those patients requiring oestrogen supplementation at the menopause and after a hysterectomy.

Treatment of oestrogen deficiency

The response to oestrogen treatment in those with specific oestrogen deficiency may be dramatic, but the response of the non-specific symptoms is more variable. Patients with a poor response to oestrogen therapy may be found to be suffering from cyclical symptoms, and these women are the ones more likely to benefit from progesterone.

Women with an intact uterus should be given oestrogen in three-weekly courses, together with a progestogen, for a minimum of 14 days to ensure that adequate cyclical bleeding occurs, thus preventing undue thickening of the endometrium, which may be a precursor to carcinoma of the body of the uterus (Studd *et al.*). Oestradiol valeate or sulphate are probably the best oestrogens to use at the menopause as ethinyloestradiol has high clotting risks and conjugated equine oestrogens have high steroidal levels. The non-steroidal oestrogens such as stilboestrol, hexaestradiol and dioenestrol are best avoided as there is a possibility that they may prove carcinogenic. Some women benefit from the oestrogen but find the progestogen causes tension and depression, in which case progesterone suppositories may be given for the last few days of each course to ensure bleeding.

Women who have had a hysterectomy and require oestrogen can have continuous medication without any fear of causing carcinogenic changes in the uterus.

If a woman complains of headaches, bloatedness or depression when the three-week course of oestrogen is stopped it suggests either that the dose was too high, or that treatment has been started too early before menopausal symptoms were present. Such patients often benefit from progesterone or progestogens for a year and are then ready for oestrogen therapy.

Contraindications for oestrogen therapy

Patients in whom oestrogens are contraindicated include the following:

1. Past history of coronary thrombosis or present history of angina.
2. History of deep-vein thrombosis or pulmonary embolism.
3. Hormone-dependent carcinoma of the breast, uterus or ovary.
4. Diabetes, kidney or liver disease.
5. Hypertension. Extra precautions are needed in those with a marked family history of hypertension, hypercholesterolaemia, ischaemic heart disease or cerebral vascular accidents.

Progestogen therapy

Progestogen therapy is valuable for use in women in whom oestrogen is contraindicated, or who develop side effects on oestrogen. In these patients, the problems of progestogens lowering the blood level of progesterone is no longer important. Progestogens are effective in stopping the flushes, preventing oesteoporosis and improving the general wellbeing. Doses of norethisterone 5–10mg may be used.

24

The sociological significance of premenstrual syndrome

World-wide evidence is accumulating to show that the effects of premenstrual syndrome are present in every aspect of a woman's life, but this does not mean in every woman's life. At times the evidence seems so universal that there is a tendency to forget that not every woman suffers to the same extent or in the same way, and that only 40–50% of the total female population are handicapped by the cyclical hormonal swings of menstruation. Studies into the sociological effect of this syndrome are likely to become more difficult and harder to interpret in future as a larger proportion of women take contraceptive pills. As explained in Chapter 10, these tend to blur the distinctive phases of the menstrual cycle and produce side effects in sufferers from premenstrual syndrome. (See Appendix for the inability to tolerate the pill by 85% of sufferers from premenstrual syndrome, although those with spasmodic dysmenorrhoea enjoy a positive benefit from the pill.) Studies into sports performance in relation to menstruation, at a teacher training college in the north of England, have already been abandoned because too high a proportion of the women students were on the pill; moreover, it was difficult to discern the motivation of that group of 18–20-year-olds who abstained. Were they ignorant, foolhardy or wise?

Effect on schoolgirls' work

The effect of the hormone fluctuations on young girls was shown in a study of 1560 weekly grades of schoolgirls during one term at a boarding school. Their work was marked in some 7–12 subjects. Each grade was compared with that of the previous week and it was noticed that the standard of school work fell below the norm by 10% during the premenstrual week in comparison with a rise above the norm of 20% during the postmenstrual week. Furthermore, this pattern of premenstrual fall and postmenstrual rise was present equally in all age groups; it occurred among girls with only one menstruation per term and those who were menstruating each month; it was equally distributed among the bright girls and the duller ones, the consistent and the inconsistent worker (Fig. 24.1) (Dalton, 1960a).

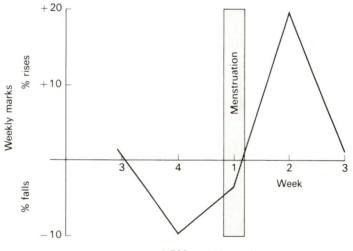

1,560 weekly grades

Fig. 24.1   Variation in schoolgirls' weekly grades with menstruation. (From Dalton K. (1960). *Br. Med. J.*; **1:**326.)

The effect of menstruation on examinations was shown in a boarding school where girls of an average age of 16 years were taking ordinary ('O') level examinations and girls of an average age of 18 years were taking advanced ('A') level school-leaving exminations. Those girls who were unfortunate enough to take examinations during their paramenstruum had fewer passes, fewer distinctions and lower average marks. It also appeared that among the 91 'O' level candidates it was those whose menstruation had a duration of six or more days who had most failures (Fig. 24.2) (Dalton, 1968).

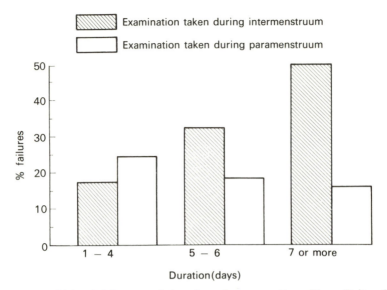

Fig. 24.2   'O' level failures and duration of menstruation. (From Dalton K. (1968). *Lancet*; **ii**:1386.)

In addition, those girls whose menstrual cycle exceeded 31 days had more failures than the girls with shorter cycles (Fig. 24.3). The effect of the stress of these examinations in altering the girls' menstrual cycle is shown in Fig. 5.1.

These fluctuations in mental ability related to menstruation are not limited to the schoolgirl, but continue throughout the menstruating years. They may be evidenced by the typist whose typing errors increase, by the secretary who notes down the wrong telephone number and by the actress who suddenly experiences difficulty in learning her part.

Effect on schoolgirls' behaviour

Further observations were made on boarding schoolgirls in respect of punishments. A total of 272 offences had been committed during the 14 days before and the 14 days after the first day of menstruation. It was found that the statistically significant

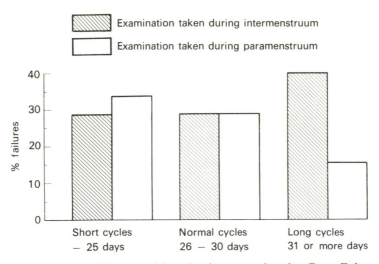

Fig. 24.3   'O' level failures and length of menstrual cycle. (From Dalton K. (1968). *Lancet*; **ii**:1386.)

figure of 29% of all offences had been committed during the first four days of menstruation, which compares with an expected incidence of 14% had there been an even distribution of offences committed during the 28 days (Fig. 24.4). Common offences were forgetfulness and unpunctuality, which may be attributed to lethargy. Indeed, a girl with a delayed judgment time is more likely to be punished for an offence because she was too slow to avoid detection (Dalton, 1960c).

Another interesting feature was that sixth form prefects aged 16–18 years, who were permitted to punish girls for misbehaviour, gave significantly more punishments during their own menstruation. Their standards of discipline tended to rise at each menstruation and then gradually fall during the cycle (Fig. 24.5). The same is true of teachers, and many a sixth-form girl will watch the day-to-day irritability or calmness of her mistress to decide when is a good moment to hand in an essay or ask a favour.

The effect of menstruation on tidiness was seen in the dormitory of a London school, where each morning the 24 boarders, aged between 10 and 14 years, received a grade A to D from the matron for the tidiness of each girl's bed and drawer. An interesting pattern resulted, showing falls in tidiness grades occurring at intervals of 21–30 days. The dates of menstruation

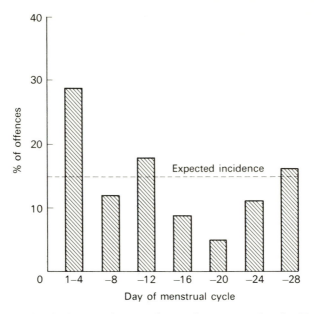

Fig. 24.4   Schoolgirls' punishments during the menstrual cycle. (From Dalton K. (1960). *Br. Med. J.*; **2**:1425.)

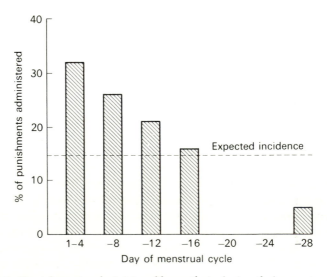

Fig. 24.5   Punishments administered by prefects during their menstrual cycle. (From Dalton K. (1960). *Br. Med. J.*; **2**:1425.)

were unknown except for girl 1; it is significant that each of her three falls in tidiness grade coincided with menstruation. The question remains, was premenstrual lethargy responsible for the carelessness of the schoolgirls before breakfast?

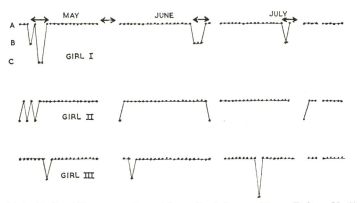

Fig. 24.6   Daily tidiness grades with cyclical drops. (From Dalton K. (1960). *Br. Med. J.*; **1**:326.)

Studies of criminal women

A study in a woman's prison published in 1961 showed that among those who had committed their offence during the previous 28 days, 49% of 156 newly committed prisoners had been sentenced for crimes committed during the paramenstruum (P=<0.001). Premenstrual syndrome of an incapacitating severity was present in 27% of these 156 prisoners, and it was found that 63% of these had committed their crimes during the paramenstruum – the time during which the triad of lethargy, irritability and depression was at its peak. In contrast, spasmodic dysmenorrhoea (Chapter 19) was present in 14% of these prisoners, and they had committed their crimes evenly throughout the menstrual cycle. During their stay in prison those who became disorderly were reported daily to the prison governor, and here again there was a high relationship between menstruation and misbehaviour (Fig. 24.7). Indeed, among those whose misbehaviour caused them to be reported more than once, 70% of offences had been committed during the paramenstruum (Dalton, 1961).

In the same London womens' prison 20 years later D'Orban and

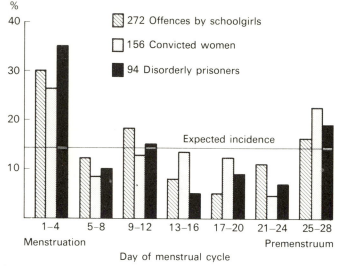

Fig. 24.7   Times of offences during menstrual cycle. (From Dalton K. (1961). *Br. Med. J.*; **2**:1752.)

Dalton (1980) (not related to the author) studied 50 women charged with crimes of violence and found that 44% had committed their offence during the paramenstruum (Fig. 24.8) and that 34% suffered from premenstrual symptoms, compared with the earlier finding of 27%, but the women with symptoms did not show any tendency to commit their offences during the paramenstruum. The authors feel that their findings cannot be accounted for by psychosocial explanations, and support the alternative hypothesis that endocrine, rather than social or psychological factors, are responsible for the association between offences of violence and the paramenstruum.

Figure 24.7 shows the close similarity in the timing of offences committed by schoolgirls, newly-convicted prisoners and disorderly ones in relation to menstruation. The hormonal changes of menstruation render the individual less amenable to discipline, more tense, and less alert so that she is more likely to be detected in her misdoings. Another aspect to be considered when schoolgirls, students or prisoners are living together in dormitories, is the possibility of menstrual synchrony occurring, which it is more likely to do when emotional experiences are shared, such as examination stress or end-of-term excitement.

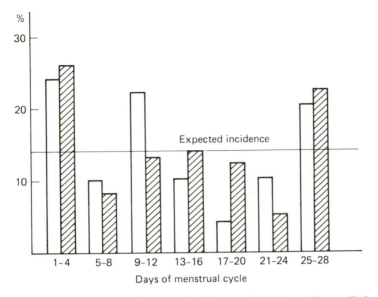

Fig. 24.8   Distribution of 50 offences of violence and 156 other offences (Dalton, 1961) during four-day periods of the menstrual cycle. (From D'Orban P.T., Dalton J. (1980). *Psychological Medicine*; **10**:353–359.)

This tendency for their menstruations to synchronise compounds the problems of the paramenstruum.

Legal implications

In 1980 two cases came before the criminal court in which women charged with manslaughter, successfully pleaded diminished responsibility due to premenstrual syndrome, and so changed British legal history. The diagnosis of the first case is fully described in Chapter 4, Figs. 3.14–3.15 (Dalton, 1980). These verdicts bring a new responsibility to the medical profession, whose task will be to ensure that the plea of premenstrual syndrome is not abused. In every case the diagnosis needs to be substantiated with incontrovertible evidence and proof that the syndrome will respond to progesterone therapy. Those few sufferers of premenstrual syndrome who experience a sudden lack of control and become aggressive or violent need help and help is available; they must not be confused with the other 99% of women who are well able to control their actions. Merely to be caught shoplifting or driving dangerously during the premenstruum is insufficient evidence for a defence of premenstrual syndrome. It is the duty of society to ensure that the genuine sufferer from premenstrual syndrome receives treatment and not a criminal record, at the same time ensuring that the malingerer does not benefit from a plea of premenstrual syndrome (Dalton, 1981).

There are certain features which characterise the criminal offences committed by sufferers of premenstrual syndrome, and which are easily recognised:

1. The woman acts alone without an accomplice.
2. The offence is not premeditated and usually comes as a surprise to those who were with her shortly before her offence.
3. The action is without apparent motive, such as stabbing one's best friend or committing arson on an unknown person's property.
4. There may be no attempt to escape detection. A woman may randomly throw a brick at a shop window, then telephone the police and wait patiently to be arrested.
5. The action may be a cri de coeur, as with the hoaxer who repeatedly makes emergency telephone calls to the police or fire station.

Among the premenstrual symptoms which may result in criminal charges are a sudden and momentary surge of uncontrollable emotions resulting in violence, confusion, amnesia, alcoholism, nymphomania and attention-seeking episodes, which represent cries for help.

The effect on industry

The cost to industry of the effect of menstruation is high. In Sweden it was estimated that 5% of absenteeism in factory, office and high school, in all communities, occurred during menstruation, while in the United Kingdom it is reckoned to be about 3% of the women at work. Among women employees using the sickbay at work, 45% do so during their paramenstruum (Fig. 24.9) (Dalton, 1964).

The effect on industry is felt most acutely where there is heavy reliance on female labour for their special skills, such as in the

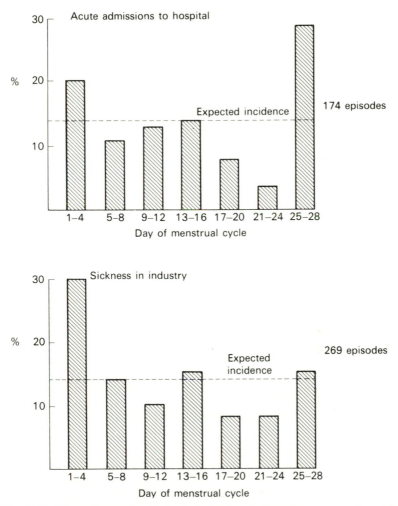

Fig. 24.9   Time of acute hospital admissions and of employees reporting sick.
(From Dalton K. (1964). *Proc. Roy. Soc. Med.*; **57:4**,262.)

clothing trade, light engineering and assembly work. Texas
Industries noted that among women employed for the assembly
of electrical components a worker's normal production rate of 100
components an hour was reduced to around 75 during the paramenstruum. In the retail and distributive trades there may be a
variety of effects ranging from errors in stocktaking and billing
to bad-tempered service to customers and breakages from

clumsiness. In the office the irritability may result in a sudden argument with the boss, the cleaner spilling her bucket of water across the room, the secretary hurling spoilt letters into the basket and a longstanding employee irrationally giving notice.

Accident proneness

In the wards of four London teaching hospitals it was noted that 52% of admissions for accidents occurred during the para-menstruum (Fig. 24.10) (Dalton, 1960b), a figure since confirmed by the United States Center for Safety Education, who pinpointed the 48 hours immediately before the onset of menstruation as the time when accidents are most likely to occur.

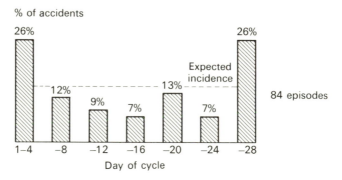

Fig. 24.10 Distribution of 84 accidents during the menstrual cycle. (From Dalton K. (1960), *Br. Med. J.*; **2**:1425.)

The significance of menstruation as a factor affecting accident proneness is clearly portrayed in the accidents on the road, in the home and factory and at sport; it is to be found equally among those performing routine daily tasks and those participating in unusual manoeuvres. Once again, one notices the increased mental and physical lethargy, the lowered judgment and increased clumsiness. The driver is liable to make irrational decisions when overtaking, she may be impatient with slow drivers and feel aggressive towards other drivers at traffic lights. During the paramenstruum her visual acuity will be decreased and she may have more difficulty at judging distances and in doing complicated tasks such as reversing.

Social workers face an increased workload when women under

their care are in the paramenstruum, for this is the time the mother is most likely to cause non-accidental injury to her children, when she may irrationally refuse entry to her home, when she is likely to quarrel with her husband, in-laws or neighbours who may report her, and when she becomes more readily intoxicated with alcohol.

Effect on morbidity

The influence of menstruation on the onset of morbidity was shown during an investigation carried out in the medical and surgical wards of a general hospital, and in the wards of an infectious fever hospital, when 49% of 174 acute admissions of women were found to have occurred during the paramenstruum (Fig. 24.9) (Dalton, 1964).

An interesting facet of the survey was the finding that viral infections tended to occur during the premenstruum, while bacterial infections predominated during menstruation. The difference may be due to the longer prodromal phase, characteristic of bacterial infection, the infection starting in the premenstruum and becoming acute during menstruation, or because bacterial infections were secondary to viral infection in the premenstruum. On the other hand, it could be related to the immunosuppressive action of progesterone.

Effects on sports

Even at leisure the woman is not free from the paramenstrual influence, as her partner at bridge may have discovered, or her opponent at chess or Scrabble may well appreciate. Sport may be affected, and in the days before our sportswomen controlled their menstruation with hormones it was possible to foretell who would be the likely winner at tennis and other small ball sports by reference to previous performances and the effect of premenstrual syndrome. The rise in intraocular pressure that occurs in the premenstruum affects the visual acuity (Dalton, 1967). Hand and arm steadiness varies during the cycle with the unsteadiness occurring during the paramenstruum; simple reaction time is not altered (Pierson & Lockhart), but judgment and mental ability are. Even a slight degree of paramenstrual dyspnoea due to engorgement of the bronchial and nasal mucosa may prove a handicap in many sports.

25

The effect of the premenstrual syndrome on the family

The linchpin of the family is the mother, so when her life becomes a misery each month and the disturbances of premenstrual syndrome recur, the consequences affect the whole family – the husband, infants, schoolchildren, teenagers, and even elderly grandparents. The tragedy is that too often it continues with cyclical regularity and no one does anything about it. In its mildest form other adults should be able to joke about premenstrual syndrome, making allowances for the temporary disturbing behaviour, but when it is severe, with symptoms causing marital stress and family suffering, specific treatment should be given.

The young infant

Children and young infants of only a few months are most sensitive to mother's changes of temperament; they find it impossible to understand the mood changes and fluctuations and may react with psychosomatic problems, such as a cough, runny nose, endless crying or vomiting. In the author's general practice mothers were asked to record the dates of their menstruation, and on a separate chart to record the days of their children's recurrent symptoms. After two or three months it was astonishing how many children's ailments reflected their difficulty in adjusting to the disturbances of mother's paramenstruum (Fig. 25.1). Even a nine-month-old girl reacted with an upper respiratory infection for three consecutive months, each one occurring during her mother's premenstruum (Dalton, 1966).

240

	Jan.	Feb.	Mar.	Apr.	May	Jun.
1						
2						
3						
4						
5						
6						
7						
8						
9						X
10						X
11						X
12						X
13						XM
14					X	XM
15					X	XM
16					X	M
17					X	
18					MX	
19			X		M	
20			X		M	
21			X	X	M	
22		X	MX	X	M	
23		X	MX	M		
24		X	M	M		
25		MX	M	M		
26		MX		M		
27		M				
28		M				
29						
30						
31						
Total						

M = mother's menstruation

X = child's colds

Male child 2 years 4 months.

Fig. 25.1 Relationship of a child's colds to mother's menstruation.

A survey of 100 mothers attending surgery because their children had coughs or colds, showed that 54% of the mothers were in their paramenstruum (Fig. 25.2). The children at risk of a surgery attendance during their mother's paramenstruum were those under two years (71%), only children (67%), those with symptoms of less than 24 hours' duration (66%) and those whose mothers were under 30 years (63%).

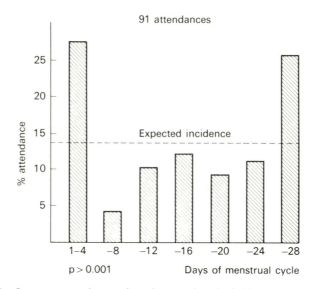

Fig. 25.2   Surgery attendance of mothers with sick children. (From Dalton K. (1969). *The Menstrual Cycle,* Penguin Books.)

There was a possibility that the general practice was biased, so the survey was repeated at the North Middlesex Hospital, a general district hospital, questioning the mothers of 100 children who had been admitted as an emergency. The result was similar; whether the admission was for an accident or an illness, 49% of the mothers were in their paramenstruum at the time of their child's admission (Fig. 25.3). Of course, if the mother is accident-prone during her paramenstruum, her action may result in an accident to either herself or to her child – for example, if she is pouring out the tea and spills it, the boiling tea may either scald her or her child, if he is standing too near (Dalton, 1970).

Tuch (1975) confirmed these findings in Los Angeles Children's Hospital. He defined the paramenstruum as the five pre-menstrual days and the first six days of the cycle, and found that children brought in by mothers in their paramenstruum were considered to be less sick, to be suffering from different types of illnesses, and to have been sick for a shorter time than children brought in by mothers in their intermenstruum.

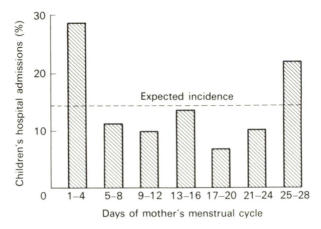

Fig. 25.3 Children's hospital admissions and mothers' menstruation. (From Dalton K. (1968). *Lancet*; ii:1386.)

Sibling jealousy misdiagnosed

It is easy to diagnose 'sibling jealousy' in an older child who has displayed symptoms of temper tantrums, enuresis or recurrent abdominal pain only since the birth of a younger sibling, but there may be another explanation. Premenstrual syndrome tends to increase in severity with age and parity, especially if the pregnancy had been complicated by pre-eclampsia or postnatal depression.

A 30-year-old mother had been 'better than ever' during her second pregnancy. She would take her son aged three years each afternoon to play on the swings or kick a football in the recreation grounds. However, following an easy labour and the delivery of a much-wanted daughter, she became severely depressed, needing psychiatric help. During the following year her son who had been dry, developed enuresis again. Of course, his sister was inevitably blamed until a chart (Fig. 25.4) showed that his bedwetting nights coincided with his mother's premenstruum. She then admitted that during the premenstruum she became too lethargic to play football or take unnecessary walks in the park and possibly even to attend to his toilet before bedtime; also, her breasts became tender and she spent her time fending him off when he wanted a good hug. Treatment of mother's premenstrual syndrome ended her son's enuresis (Dalton, 1977).

	Jul.	Aug.	Sep.	Oct.	Nov.	Dec.
1						
2					X	
3					M	
4					M	
5				X	M	
6					M	
7				X	M	
8					M	
9				M		
10				M		
11				M		
12				M		
13				M		
14			X	M		
15			M	M		
16			M			
17			M			
18			M			
19			M			
20		X	M			
21			M			
22		M	M			
23		M				
24		M				
25		M				
26		M				
27		M				
28		M				
29		M				
30						
31						
Total						

M = Mother's menstruation
X = Child's enuresis

Fig. 25.4   Enuresis chart and mother's menstruation.

Non-accidental injury

The most tragic presentation of premenstrual syndrome is when the mother has a sudden aggressive outburst and in an irrational hysterical attack batters her baby. When non-accidental injury is suspected in an apparently loving mother one of the most important questions to ask is the date of her last menstruation.

A social worker's report on a 35-year-old mother of two children read: "During the last premenstruum her youngest daughter, aged 18 months, was screaming and would not stop. Patient was very irritated by this and picked her up and squeezed her – this started a circle of louder screaming and a harder squeezing until patient 'heard something crack'. She was immediately frightened and threw the child on the floor and sat crying on a chair. When more composed she examined the child and took her to the doctor.'

A 27-year-old housewife explained; 'I was teaching my five-year-old daughter to weave – she wasn't attending – she kept looking out of the window – I shouted at her – she started trembling – then I couldn't help it I hit her good and truly. It was only afterwards I realised I had started menstruating.'

Both these women were treated with progesterone and their aggression stopped.

The schoolchild

When the child goes to school it may be obvious to teachers from a glance at the lateness register or absentee list that the mother is having monthly difficulties. School doctors should be informed of such warning signs. It was noticed that a 10-year-old girl's name repeatedly appeared on the absent list at the beginning of each month. When the mother attended a few days later it transpired that she had recurrent asthma which necessitated bed rest and the daughter was kept at home to answer the door. How much better to treat the mother's premenstrual asthma rather than let the child's education suffer.

On a mother's lethargic premenstrual days she is liable to send the children off on errands and then scold them for buying items that are too expensive, or for getting the wrong change. She may be too tired to attend school concerts or parents' evenings when they occur in the paramenstruum.

Teenagers' problems

Unfortunately, due to the average age differences, for many families, the teenage years of the children coincide with a worsening of premenstrual syndrome during the premenopausal phase of the mother. When premenstrual tension gets worse teenagers find it difficult to make contact with mother, never being sure of her reaction beforehand, or they may turn aside with the comment, 'She's in one of her moods – don't ask her today.'

Daughters are more likely to understand the mood changes and may indeed have personal experience. It is important to discuss the problem openly with teenagers of both sexes, explaining to them that many of the quarrels with their friends and their unexpected tears may well be due to the changes in hormonal levels.

Menstrual synchrony

With mother and daughter living closely together there is the possibility of menstrual synchrony occurring, so exacerbating any disharmony in the household during the paramenstruum (McClinton).

One mother wrote about her daughter who was receiving treatment for premenstrual irritability and food cravings. 'Some cakes and biscuits disappeared on Sunday. It was all too much for me and I burst in tears. This in turn upset my husband, who went and found my daughter in her bedroom and gave her a good thrashing. At midnight we discovered she was missing. She had spent the night with friends.' Both mother and daughter started menstruating that same day.

The grandparents

The elderly grandparents may also be the butt of their daughter's jaded premenstrual moods, at which time continual complaints are made of their eating and sleeping habits or their failure to follow simple instructions. In general practice the doctor watches as the elderly parent gradually becomes more senile and helpless, and stands by ready to offer help and social services as they are needed. But it is interesting how suddenly – and it always is suddenly and with great urgency – the request is made for the elderly relative to be moved away. The daughter can no longer cope – it is all too much for her. At great length and in the finest detail she will tell of all the difficulties. If at this moment it is possible to ask her, it is usual to find that the caring relative is in her paramenstruum and her ability to care and to love has temporarily disappeared, although it will return in the postmenstruum. More than one husband has arranged for help in the home for one week each month, rather than one day each week, in order to prepare for the difficulties of the paramenstruum.

The husband

The wise husband knows that when his wife wakes up 'a changed personality' it is one of those days when he must treat her with care or else her irrational wrath will burst upon him.

To be married to a sufferer of severe premenstrual syndrome calls forth qualities of understanding, flexibility and leadership. The husband needs to be aware of the fluctuations of mood during the paramenstruum and have confidence that normality will be resumed once the postmenstruum is reached. He needs to be ready to step into the breach and assume control at awkward moments. Most of all, he must realise that stress will increase the severity of her symptoms and also that long spells without food may have disastrous consequences and can always be avoided.

One survey showed that the husband's late arrival at work was a reflection of the time of his wife's cycle. They both failed to get up with the alarm, they quarrelled over breakfast, which consequently took longer, and then the sandwiches weren't ready!

A door-to-door salesman was referred for treatment after his employers noticed that one week in four his sales record was abysmal and his commission practically nil. By consultation with his wife's diary it became apparent that the bad weeks corresponded in each instance with his wife's paramenstruum. During the interview the husband spoke of his wife's changed personality on those days, how she became 'impatient and dogmatic'. When she had received progesterone treatment, the husband returned saying she was now 'like the woman I married'.

One husband realised that if they discussed their household budget and possible economies during the paramenstruum no agreement could be reached. He solved the problem by asking the bank manager to send the statements at carefully chosen dates when his wife was in her postmenstruum and would be reasonable and amenable to suggestions.

Henderson of Melbourne has shown that the husband's basal temperature curve is related to that of his wife and that both have a characteristic ovulation drop followed by a rise in temperature, although this does not occur when the woman is on the contraceptive pill nor among men living alone.

The young child is the most sensitive barometer of the approaching storms and tempests foreshadowed by the mother's premenstrual pattern. The husband and older children come next and it is important that their ability to diagnose the condition is used to the full. Doctors should always be ready to listen to the husband's story.

26

A glimpse of the future

By the time this book is published it will be 36 years since Dr Raymond Greene first introduced the author to progesterone for the treatment of her premenstrual migraine and the rapidly developing symptoms of premenstrual syndrome. Three months later, as a general practitioner, the first case of premenstrual asthma received progesterone treatment. Now, tens of thousands of well-treated premenstrual syndrome patients later, it might be expected that the disease and its treatment would be fully understood by the medical world and this book would no longer be necessary. But, such is the capriciousness and reserve of the medical and psychological disciplines, that we are far from that ideal state.

Most psychologists and psychiatrists can see premenstrual syndrome only as a behavioural condition and, as the psychologists rarely do a physical examination of the patient, they are unaware of the physical aspects of the disease.

All is not gloom, however, for among the endocrinologists there are groups of workers who, in seeking to understand the actions and interactions of the reproductive hormones, are beginning to explain the conundrums which are produced by premenstrual syndrome. Exciting possibilities are emerging from the work on endorphins, inhibin, the pineal secretions and *in vitro* fertilisation. In this field the seeds are germinating for the full understanding of the vital role of progesterone in the hormonal jungle.

It is already apparent that premenstrual syndrome, luteal phase defect, pre-eclampsia and postnatal depression are all part of the same progesterone deficiency syndrome although as more becomes known progesterone deficiency may turn out to be but a stage in the train of other hormonal defects which eventually it will be possible to resolve.

There is little doubt that these are hereditary diseases and therefore a genetic fault may eventually be detected which genetic engineering could probably correct, but this is all conjecture and rests with the research workers in these topics.

Meanwhile, practical hope comes from the knowledge that more and more family doctors are now learning to recognise, diagnose and treat with progesterone, as and where it is properly required. About 10% of British general practitioners are waking up to an appreciation of the remarkable response of well-diagnosed premenstrual syndrome to progesterone therapy.

Other steps towards that better future have been made with the recognition of those young girls who are once-a-month nymphomaniacs, regularly running away from home to satisfy their uncontrollable libido. These, too, can now be successfully treated and restored to normality. Then there is the realisation of the immunosuppressive property of progesterone and the recognition that its use in all the diseases mentioned above is prophylactic, which assures us that if we use it in this way pre-eclampsia and postnatal depression will begin to disappear like an 'icicle in the sun'.

The saving this would provide in the high cost of hospitalisation, time lost in industry, family and social unhappiness and, indeed, as we are now realising, the misery of women being labelled criminals and sent to prison for those diagnosable and treatable episodes of loss of control that bring them into conflict with the law, is incalculable. But even brighter is the future for those with luteal phase defect who may now look forward to bearing the child that they desire.

All this is possible – once the old habits and shibboleths can be shed and we can look with clear, unprejudiced eyes at the evidence which has now been placed before us.

Appendix

The medical records were analysed of all women, personally seen by the author during 1982, who were currently receiving, or had received progesterone therapy in the previous 35 years. All patients had been referred to the author by another doctor, almost invariably by the patient's general practitioner, who was also responsible for prescribing the progesterone.

Two research assistants scrutinised the files of 2180 patients, and extracted the details of 1274 (58%) women, who had received progesterone for the reasons shown in Table 27.1.

Premenstrual syndrome

The diagnosis had been confirmed by a three month menstrual chart and throughout treatment the patient continued to maintain a record on her chart, a duplicate of which was kept in her file to monitor progress. Tables 27.2 and 27.3 show the age and parity of the 1095 women, who received progesterone for premenstrual syndrome.

Table 27.4 shows the presenting symptoms in premenstrual syndrome at that first visit and Table 27.5 shows other premenstrual symptoms which were spontaneously mentioned at that interview. The preponderance of psychological symptoms is evident in both tables. Premenstrual anxiety and alcohol excess are more frequent symptoms among parous, compared with nulliparous women, while criminal acts and skin lesions predominate in nulliparous women. The time of onset of premenstrual syndrome is linked to hormonal events by 87% of women. Similarly, 182 women (86%) whose symptoms had increased in severity, linked it to hormonal events (Table 27.7). This was more marked among parous women. The non-hormonal events noted included marriage, bereavement, separation, moving home, glandular fever, mumps and immigration.

The time of onset and of increased severity was noted to follow

251

Table 27.1

Reasons for progesterone therapy

Premenstrual syndrome		1095
Posthysterectomy premenstrual syndrome		126
Hysterectomy	74	
Hysterectomy and unilateral oophorectomy	17	
Hysterectomy and bilateral oophorectomy	35	
Prophylaxis of postnatal depression		32
Defective luteal phase		13
Others: pregnancy	3	7
hirsute	2	
amenorrhoea	2	
	Total	1273

Table 27.2

Age and parity at first visit of premenstrual syndrome patients

Age	Nulliparous		Parous		Total	
years	n	%	n	%	n	%
−20	59	100%	–	–	59	5%
−25	52	63%	31	37%	83	8%
−30	61	41%	87	59%	148	13%
−35	61	19%	252	81%	313	29%
−40	47	19%	200	81%	247	22%
−45	30	22%	104	78%	134	12%
−50	11	13%	72	87%	83	8%
+50	5	18%	23	82%	28	3%
Total	326	30%	769	70%	1095	100%

postnatal depression in 9% (Tables 27.6 & 27.7). Bilateral tubal ligation had been performed on 11% of the women.

The incidence of side-effects from oral contraceptives in 614 pill takers with premenstrual syndrome (Table 27.8) reveals that the incidence rises with age, and is more marked in parous women. Depression and headache are more common in parous women, while weight gain is more common in nulliparous women (Table 27.9).

Table 27.3

Parity of premenstrual syndrome patients before treatment

Fullterm pregnancies	n	%
None	326	30
One	221	20
Two	369	34
Three	144	13
Four or more	35	3
Abortions		
None	763	70
One	234	22
Two	58	5
Three	25	2
Four or more	15	1
After treatment		
Fullterm pregnancies	70	61
Spontaneous abortions	9	8
Terminations of pregnancy	10	9
Currently pregnant	26	22
Total	115	100

Table 27.4

Presenting symptom in premenstrual syndrome

n	Nulliparous	Parous	Total
	326	769	1095
	%	%	%
Tension (depression, irritability and lethargy)	76	71	73
Headache/migraine	21	22	20
Epilepsy	4	2	3
Psychosis	2	2	2
Asthma	2	1	1
Eye	–	1	0.5
Urinary	1	1	0.5
Skin	–	–	–
ENT	–	–	–

Table 27.5

Other premenstrual symptoms in premenstrual syndrome

	Nulliparous		Parous		Total	
	n=326		n=769		n=1095	
	n	%	n	%	n	%
Bloatedness	107	33	256	33	364	33
Headache	78	24	199	26	277	25
Breast tenderness	69	21	169	22	238	22
Depression	61	19	110	14	171	16
Irritability	39	12	94	12	133	12
Anxiety/panics	26*	8	105*	14	131	12
Tiredness	31	9	62	8	93	8
Suicidal	25	8	52	7	77	7
Food cravings	20	6	40	5	60	5
Criminal acts	22*	6	16*	2	38	3
Vertigo	12	3	26	3	38	3
Alcohol	14*	4	18*	2	32	3
Skin	15*	4	10*	3	25	3
Ear, nose and throat	9	2	14	2	23	2
Eye	4	1	13	2	17	2
Urinary	3	1	5	1	8	1
Asthma	1	–	6	1	7	1

* = Probability <0.05.

A previous history of amenorrhoea (14%) was noted among nulliparous women under 35 years (Table 27.10).

The incidence of previous pre-eclampsia and postnatal depression in 769 parous women with premenstrual syndrome is shown in Table 27.11.

Chapter 21 gives the incidence of postnatal depression, severe enough to require medical attention, as between 7–14%, however, this present analysis shows an overall figure of postnatal depression of 59% rising to 71% for the under twenty-fives.

The previous medication prescribed for premenstrual syndrome (Table 27.12) shows interesting differences in relation to age, tranquillisers being prescribed to 29% in those over 35 years, and antidepressants most frequently to the 26–35 age group. Oral contraceptives are tried more often by the younger groups;

Table 27.6

Time of onset of premenstrual syndrome

	Nulliparous	Parous	Total
n	326	769	1095
	%	%	%
Puberty	57	26	32
After abortion	6	–	–
After pregnancy	–	40	33
Postnatal depression	–	12	9
Oral contraceptives	10	7	8
Amenorrhoea	9	1	3
Sterilisation	2	3	3
Oophorectomy	3	–	1
Hormonal event	84	89	87
Non-hormonal event	10	8	9
Don't know	6	3	4

Table 27.7

Time of increased severity of premenstrual syndrome

	Nulliparous	Parous	Total
n	25	157	182
	%	%	%
After abortion	24	–	3
After pregnancy	–	57	49
Postnatal depression	4	11	9
Oral contraceptives	24	8	10
Amenorrhoea	12	1	2
Sterilisation	4	12	11
Hormonal event	68	89	86
Non-hormonal event	32	11	14

Table 27.8

Side-effects of oral contraceptives in premenstrual syndrome
by age and parity

Age/Years	Nulliparous	Parous	Total
	side-effects %	side-effects %	side-effects %
n Pill takers	144	470	614
Under 25	65	81	70
35	77	85	84
45	77	91	89
Over 45	100	88	88
Total	74	88	85

Table 27.9

Side-effects from oral contraceptives in premenstrual syndrome

	Nulliparous	Parous	Total
Total Pill takers	144	470	614
	%	%	%
Depression	15	23	21
Headache	16	21	20
Weight gain	17	12	13
Nausea	10	10	10
Increased tension	8	7	7
Bloatedness	5	6	5
Loss of libido	5	4	4
Breast tenderness	3	3	3

Table 27.10

Incidence of previous amenorrhoea in premenstrual syndrome

Age/Years	Nulliparous		Parous		Total	
	Total in group n	amen- orrhoea %	Total in group n	amen- orrhoea %	Total in group n	amen- orrhoea %
Under 25	111	13	31	3	142	11
35	122	15	339	3	461	6
45	77	5	304	3	381	4
Over 45	16	–	95	–	111	–
	326	11	769	3	1095	7

Table 27.11

Incidence of previous pre-eclampsia and postnatal depression
in premenstrual syndrome

Age/Years	Total in group	% Pre-eclampsia	% Postnatal depression
Under 25	31	13	71
35	339	15	69
45	304	16	54
Over 45	95	7	41
Total	769	14	59

8% compared with the older group (2%); in contrast analgesics are prescribed more frequently to the oldest group (9%). There is then an age related reduction in the frequency until only 3% receive analgesics in the youngest group.

Table 27.13 shows that at their last visit 86% were receiving progesterone suppositories, 6% injections, 2% an implant and 6% had discontinued progesterone treatment. The most frequent dosage was 400mg twice daily (33%) and only 6% received less than 400mg daily. The day of starting progesterone is shown in Table 27.14, revealing that progesterone was started on Day 14

Table 27.12

Previous medication for premenstrual syndrome in relation to age

Age/Years	Under 25	− 35	− 45	Over 45	Total
n	142	461	381	111	1096
	%	%	%	%	%
Tranquillisers	24	25	29	29	27
Antidepressants	20	27	19	21	23
Progestogens	15	19	25	19	20
Diuretics	8	10	14	14	11
Pyridoxine	7	9	14	13	11
Analgesics	3	4	6	9	5
Oral contraceptives	8	6	4	2	5
Oestrogen	1	2	3	16	4
Hormone preparations	–	2	3	12	3
Prostoglandin inhibitors	1	2	2	1	2
Bromocriptine	–	1	2	–	1

Table 27.13

Daily dosage of progesterone at last visit

	Nulliparous	Parous	Total
n	326	769	1096
	%	%	%
Suppositories/mg:			
100 × 1	2	2	2
200 × 1	6	3	4
400 × 1	27	13	17
400 × 2	31	34	33
400 × 3	13	22	20
400 × 4	5	10	8
Over 400 × 4	2	2	2
Injections/mg:			
50	2	2	2
100	3	4	4
Implant	2	3	2
Discontinued	7	5	6

Table 27.14

Day of starting progesterone at last visit

	Nulliparous	Parous	Total
n	326	769	1095
	%	%	%
Days 8–9	8	6	6
10–	1	2	2
12–	5	8	6
14–	45	53	51
16–	7	5	6
18–	7	2	3
20–	3	1	2
22–	–	1	1
When necessary	3	1	2
Continuous	14	16	15
Discontinued	7	5	6

Table 27.15

Years since progesterone therapy started

Year treatment started	n	Years of supervision
1982	(275)*	–
1981–78	595	1220
1977–73	139	725
1972–68	55	607
1967–63	13	214
1962–58	4	87
1957–53	5	134
1952–48	9	380
Total	820	3367

* Excluding less than 12 months

in 51%, and was given continuously in 15% (including by implantation).

Table 27.15 shows that 820 women with premenstrual syndrome have, since starting progesterone treatment, been supervised for a total of 3367 years. The total duration of progesterone treatment was 2797 years (Table 27.16), thus there have been 570 years of post-therapeutic surveillance, and the average duration of therapy was 5.25 years.

Concern is frequently proclaimed in regard to the effect of long-term therapy of the natural hormone progesterone. The patients' records have been examined in respect of malignancy and diabetes (Table 27.17). There have been no known instances of cardiovascular disease developing during or after treatment in the 1095 patients. The family history is probably an understatement, many were ignorant of the cause of death of their parents, which may have occurred during their childhood or abroad. One woman developed diabetes 8 years after stopping progesterone therapy.

Certain symptom groups were analysed separately (Table 27.18). It was noted that among those presenting with headache the incidence increased with age, but was unrelated to parity under 45 years (Table 27.18).

Among the 31 premenstrual epileptics (Table 27.19) it was noted that there was a high incidence of irritability, depression and headaches preceding the epileptic attacks which is in marked contrast to the 13 premenstrual asthmatics, whose attacks are not preceded by depression or headaches. This may be taken as further confirmation of the suggestion (Chapter 20) that a premenstrual epileptic attack represents a late stage of premenstrual syndrome in the same way as an eclamptic fit represents a late stage of pre-eclampsia. In other respects the epileptic resembles the findings in premenstrual syndrome, i.e. 81% unable to tolerate the pill, 42% incidence of postnatal depression and 81% have the onset after a hormonal event.

The 13 asthmatics, otherwise resembled the rest of the series except that there were more nulliparous women (54%). Furthermore, although there were 115 pregnancies during the surveillance period of the series, none of the asthmatic group became pregnant.

There were 22 psychotics, who would become deluded, hallucinated or confused for a few days premenstrually and then spontaneously revert to normal in the postmenstruum. In all

Table 27.16

Duration of progesterone therapy for premenstrual syndrome

Years	*n*	*Treated years*
Less than 1 year	(563)*	–
1–5	373	1091
6–10	112	872
11–15	32	511
16–20	8	137
21–25	2	46
Over 25	5	140
Total	532	2797

* Excluding less than 12 months

Table 27.17

Incidence of disease in family and before, during and after progesterone therapy in premenstrual syndrome

n=1095

	Family history	*Progesterone therapy* *Before*	*During*	*After*
Diabetes	24	4	–	1*
Carcinoma				
Breast	13	1	1	–
Cervix-in-situ	–	6	1	–
Ovary	1	1	–	–
Uterus	8	–	–	–
Lung	12	–	–	–
Other	23	–	–	–
Total	57 (5%)	6	2	–
Benign breast pathology	?	25	4	–
Benign ovarian cyst	?	12	–	–
Hysterectomy fibroids 5, prolapse 2	?	n/a	7	–

* Developed diabetes 8 years later.

Table 27.18

Premenstrual headache related to age and parity

	Nulliparous	*Parous*	*Total*
n	*326*	*769*	*1095*
	%	%	%
Under 35	16	17	16
36–45	28	25	26
Over 45	44	34	35
Total	21	22	22

Table 27.19

Premenstrual symptoms in premenstrual epilepsy and asthma

	Epilepsy	*Asthma*	*Premenstrual syndrome*
n	*31*	*13*	*1095*
	%	%	%
Irritability	68	46	45
Depression	68	15	54
Tiredness	42	54	39
Headache	42	15	25
Bloatedness	38	31	33

but one of the women the onset had followed a hormonal event, e.g. menarche 5, pill 2, childbirth 11. This group was characterised by the very high incidence of postnatal depression (15 of 16 parous women) and their intolerance of the pill (100%). Their response to progesterone therapy was excellent (Table 27.20).

There were 38 women who suffered from premenstrual syndrome, who had committed criminal acts during the premenstruum. Their offences are shown in Table 27.21. They differed from the other 68 women who stated they were violent during the premenstruum, as the offenders tended to damage themselves or other persons, rather than property (Table 27.22). They were also compared with women who had premenstrual alcoholism, as

Table 27.20

Characteristics of premenstrual psychosis

	n=22 n	%
Age/Years		
Under 25	3	13
35	14	63
Over 35	5	24
Nulliparous	6	27
Parous	16	73
Onset		
Puberty	5	24
Pill	2	9
Amenorrhoea	3	13
Postnatal depression	11	50
Non-hormonal event	1	4
Pre-eclampsia	3/16	19
Postnatal depression	15/16	94
Side-effects on pill	10/10	100

Table 27.21

Offences committed by women with premenstrual syndrome

	n=38
Assault to person	20
Arson	7
Damage to property	6
Theft	6
Alcohol	6
Disorderly conduct	4
Beyond parental control: school truancy 2 nymphomania 2	4
Hoax phone calls	3
Drugs	3
Homicide	2

Table 27.22

Assault to person and property by offenders and violent women

	Offenders	Violence
n	38	68
	%	%
Assault to person	53	11
police	11	–
child	16	5
other	12	6
Damage to property	34	94

shown in Table 27.23. The offenders were younger and more prone to parasuicides and self-mutilation. As the offenders were all under 45 years they were compared with the 984 premenstrual syndrome women under 45 years. The offenders resembled the rest of the series in their inability to tolerate the pill and their high incidence of postnatal depression.

Posthysterectomy premenstrual syndrome

There were 126 women seen in 1982 who had posthysterectomy premenstrual syndrome confirmed by a three month menstrual chart, and who received progesterone therapy. The age and parity distribution is shown in Table 27.24, and the presenting symptoms in Table 27.25. It is interesting that again headaches are more frequent among parous, compared with nulliparous women. The incidence of carcinoma in the family and in patients before progesterone therapy is shown in Table 27.26. There were no cases of disease during or after treatment. The incidence of carcinoma in the family (16%) was higher in these post-hysterectomy women than in those with premenstrual syndrome (5%) and there was also a higher incidence of benign breast pathology in posthysterectomy women (9%) compared with others (3%).

Posthysterectomy premenstrual syndrome responds well to progesterone implantation and was given to 28% of women (Table 27.27).

Table 27.23

Incidence of age, parasuicide and self-mutilation in offenders

	Offenders	Alcoholics	Violent	PMS series
n	38 %	32 %	66 %	984 %
Under 25 years	53	–	9	14
26–35	37	39	45	47
36–45	10	61	46	39
Parasuicide	37	25	17	6
Self-mutilation	13	–	–	0.1

Table 27.24

Age and parity of posthysterectomy premenstrual syndrome

	Hysterectomy	Hysterectomy and unilateral oophorectomy	Hysterectomy and/or bilateral oophorectomy	Total
n	74	17	35	126
				%
Under 35 years	16	2	7	20
36–45 years	25	11	19	43
Over 45 years	33	4	9	7
Nulliparous	8	2	8	14
Parous	66	55	27	86

Table 27.25

Presenting symptoms in posthysterectomy premenstrual syndrome

	Nulliparous	Parous	Total
n	18	108	126
	%	%	%
Tension	78	67	70
Headache	17	27	25
Bloatedness	–	2	2
Breast tenderness	–	2	–
Urinary	5	1	2
Ear, nose and throat	–	1	1

Table 27.26

Incidence of disease in family, and before progesterone therapy in posthysterectomy premenstrual syndrome

	n=126	
	Family history	Before treatment
Carcinoma		
Uterus	2	2
Breast	–	1
Lung	1	–
Other	17	–
Total	20 (16%)	3
Benign breast pathology	?	11 (9%)
Benign ovarian cyst	?	8

The 126 posthysterectomy women have been under observation for 405 years (Table 27.28) including 300 years of progesterone treatment (Table 27.29) and to date no long-term side-effects have been observed.

Defective luteal phase

The success of progesterone therapy in defective luteal phase is demonstrated in the 13 women seen in 1982. Before treatment they had 2 live births and 19 abortions, whereas after treatment they had 15 live births and one abortion (Table 27.30). Treatment was given from 2 days after ovulation and continued until no pregnancy symptoms were present. The dose of progesterone is shown in Table 27.31.

Progesterone prophylaxis for postnatal depression

In 1982 progesterone prophylaxis was offered to 36 women, who had previously suffered from postnatal depression (Table 27.32). In two women the obstetricians did not co-operate and the mothers developed postnatal depression. Those who received prophylactic treatment avoided any recurrence. The time of progesterone therapy in relation to pregnancy is shown in Table 27.33.

Table 27.27

The optimum dose of progesterone in posthysterectomy
premenstrual syndrome

	n=126
Daily dose	
	%
Suppositories	
200mg	2
400mg × 1	14
400mg × 2	25
400mg × 3	14
400mg × 4	6
Injections	
100mg	4
Implant	28
Discontinued	7

Table 27.28

Years since progesterone therapy started in posthysterectomy
premenstrual syndrome

Year treatment started	n=126 n	Years of supervision
1982	(42)*	*excluded*
81–78	58	191
77–73	24	173
1966	1	17
1959	1	24
Total	84	405

* Excluding less than 12 months

Table 27.29

Duration of progesterone therapy in posthysterectomy premenstrual syndrome

Years	n	Treated years
Less than 1 year	(62)*	excluded
1–5	46	151
6–10	16	111
Over 10 years	2	38
Total	126	300

* Excluding less than 12 months

Table 27.30

Parity before and after progesterone therapy in 13 women with defective luteal phase

	Before treatment	After treatment
Fullterm pregnancies		
None	11	2
One	2	7
Two	–	4
Total live births	2	15
Abortions		
None	5	12
One	3	1
Two	2	–
Three	1	–
Four	1	–
Five	1	–
Total abortions	19	1

Table 27.31

Progesterone dosage in defective luteal phase

Daily dosage	$n=13$
Suppositories	
400mg × 1	2
400mg × 2	5
400mg × 3	1
400mg × 4	1
Injections	
100mg	3

Table 27.32

Prophylactic progesterone for postnatal depression

	Postnatal depression	Normal puerpium	Total
		$n=36$	
Previous pregnancies	44	7	51
Prophylaxis arranged Treatment given	–	34	34
Obstetrician refused to give treatment	2	–	2

Table 27.33

Time of progesterone therapy in respect of pregnancy

	Stopped before pregnancy	During pregnancy	Prophylaxis for postnatal depression	Established postnatal depression	Total
Currently pregnant	–	20	–	–	20
Fullterm pregnancy	9	37	36	26	108
Spontaneous abortion	3	6	–	–	9
Termination of pregnancy	4	1	1	–	6
Total	16	64	37	26	143

References

Chapter 1

Allen W.M. (1932). *J. Biol. Chem.*; **98**, 591–605.
Bennett F.O. (1939). *N.Z. Med. J.*; **38**, Obstet. Gynec. Sect. 11.
Marsden G.E. (1937). *Brit. Med. J.*; **2**, 1221.
McMann W. (1938). *Va. Med. Mon.*; **65**, 676.
Paterson S. (1938–9). *Trans. Edin. Soc.*; **98**, 49.
Swyer G.I.M., Daley D. (1953). *Brit. Med. J.*; **1**, 1073.
Young J. (1937). *Brit. Med. J.*; **1**, 953.

Chapter 2

Dalton K. (1959). *Brit. Med. J.*; **1**, 148.
Dalton K. (1960). *ibid*; **2**, 1307.
Dalton K. (1960). *ibid*; **2**, 1425.
Dalton K. (1960). *ibid*; **2**, 1647.
Dalton K. (1961). *ibid*; **2**, 1752.
Dalton K. (1964). *Proc. Roy. Soc. Med.*; **57**, 4, 262.
Friedman R.C. (1982). *Behaviour and the Menstrual Cycle*, Marcel Dekker Inc., New York and Basel.
Greene R., Dalton K. (1953). *Brit. Med. J.*; **1**, 1007.
Gregory B.A. (1957). *J. Psychosom. Res.*; **2**, 61.
Reid R.L., Yen S.S.C. (1981). *Amer. J. Obstet. Gynecol.*; **139**, 1, 25–102.
Tonks C.M., Rack P.H., Rose M.J. (1968). *J. Psychosom. Res.*; **2**, 319.

Chapter 3

Aitken R.C.B. (1969). *Proc. R. Soc. Med.*; **62**, 989–993.
Corner G.W. (1952). *Brit. Med. J.*; **2**, 403.
Dalton K. (1954). *Brit. Med. J.*; **2**, 1071.
Dalton K. (1973). *J. Roy. Coll. Gen. Pract.*; **23**, 97.
Dalton K. (1980). *Lancet;* ii, 1070–1071.
Dalton K. (1980). *Depression After Childbirth;* Oxford University Press, Oxford.
Dalton K. (1981). *Brit. J. Psychiatry;* **136**, 199.
Dalton K. (1982). *Behaviour and Menstrual Cycle*, Chapter 11, Ed. Friedman R.C., Marcel Dekker Inc., New York.
Dalton M.E. (1981). *Postrgard. Med. J.*; **57**, 560–561.
Dalton M.E. (1984). *J. Ster. Biochem.;* Jan.
Devi S.P., Rao A.V. (1972). *Indian J. Psychiat.*; **14**, 375–379.

Gray L.A. (1941). *Sth. Med. J.;* **34**, 1004.
Hart R.D. (1960). *Brit. Med. J.;* **1**, 1023–1024.
Iqbal M.J., Johnston M. (1977). *J. Ster. Biochem.;* 977.
Israel S.L. (1938). *J. Amer. Med. Ass.;* **110**, 1721–1723.
Moos R.H. (1968). *Psychosom. Med.;* **30**, 853–867.
Moos R.H. (1969). *Amer. J. Obstet. Gynecol.;* **103**, 390–402.
Parlee M.B. (1973). *Psychol. Bull.;* **80**, **6**, 454–465.
Radwanska E., Berger G.S., Hammond J. (1979). *Obstet. Gynec.;* **54**, 789–792.
Sampson G.A. (1979). *Br. J. Psych.;* **135**, 209–215.
Sampson G.A., Jenner F.A. (1977). *Br. J. Psych.;* **103**, 265–271.
Shader R.I., Di Mascio A., Harmatz J. (1968). *Pscyhosomat.;* **9**, **1**, 197–198.
Smith S., Sauder C. (1969). *Psychosomat. Med.;* **31**, **4**, 281.

Chapter 4

Dalton K. (1981). *Neuropharmacology;* **20**, 1267–1269.

Chapter 5

Appleby B.P. (1960). *Brit. Med. J.;* **1**, 391.
Billig H.E., Spaulding C.A. (1947). *Ind. Med.;* **16**, 336.
Bruce J., Russell G.F.M. (1962). *Lancet;* **ii**, 267.
Chesley H. (1957). *Amer. J. Obstet. Gynec.;* **74**, 582.
Dalton K. (1954). *Brit. Med. J.;* **2**, 1071.
Dalton K. (1964). *Proc. Roy. Soc. Med.;* **57**, **4**, 18.
Dalton K. (1967). *Brit. J. Ophthal.;* **51**, 10, 692.
Dalton K. (1968). *Lancet;* **ii**, 1386.
Fortin J.N., Wittkower E.D., Kalz F. (1958). *Canad. Med. Ass.;* **79**, 978.
Klein I., Carey J. (1957). *Amer. J. Obstet. Gynec.;* **74**, 956.
Lamb, W.M., Ullett G.A., Masters W.H., Robinson D.E. (1953). *Amer. J. Psychiat.;* **109**, 840.
Okey R., Stewart D. (1932–33). *J. Biol. Chem.;* **99**, 717.
Rothchild I. (1983). *Progesterone and Progestins*, Ed. Bardin C.W., Milgram E. and Mauvais-Jarvis P., Raven Press, New York, 219–230.

Chapter 6

Abramowitz E.S., Baker A.H., Fleischer S.F. (1982). *Amer. J. Psych.;* **139**, **4**, 475–478.
Belfer M.L., Carroll M. (1971). *Arch. Gen. Psychiat.;* **25**, 540.
Billig H.E. (1953). *Internat. Rec. Med.;* **11**, 166, 487.
Dalton K. (1959). *Brit. Med. J.;* **1**, 148–149.
Dalton K. (1964). *Premenstrual Syndrome*, William Heinemann Medical Books, London.
Dalton K. (1982). Evidence submitted to the FDA Washington, Feb.
Greene R., Dalton K. (1953). *Brit. Med. J.;* **1**, 1007.
Gregory B.A. (1957). *J. Psychosom. Res.;* **2**, 61.
Hart R.D. (1960). *Brit. Med. J.;* **1**, 1023.
Israel S.L. (1938). *J. Amer. Med. A;* **110**, 1721.

MacKinnon P.C.B., Mackinnon I.L. (1956). *Brit. Med. J.;* **1**, 555.
Mandell A.J., Mandell M.P. (1967). *J. Amer. Med. A.;* **200**, **9**, 792.
McCance R.A., Luff M.C., Widdowson E. (1937). *J. Hyg. (London);* **37**, 571–611.
Pollitt J. (1977). *Proc. Roy. Soc. Med.;* **70**, 145–148.
Ribeiro A.L. (1962). *Brit. Med. J.;* **1**, 640.
Wetzel R.D, McClure J.N. (1972). *Comprehensive Psych.;* **13**, **4**, 369.

Chapter 7

Billig H.E., Spaulding C.A. (1947). *Ind. Med.;* **16**, 336.
Brush M.G., Watson M., Taylor R.W. (1980). *Practitioner;* **224**, 852–855.
Clarkson B., Thomspon D., Horwigh W., Lucky E.H. (1960). *J. Amer. Med. Ass.;* **29**, 193.
Czaja J.A. (1975). *Physio. & Behaviour;* **14**, 579–587.
Dalton K. (1954). *Brit. Med. J.;* **2**, 1071.
Dalton K. (1955). *Proc. Roy. Soc. Med.;* **48**, **5**, 337.
Dalton K. (1967). *Brit. J. Ophthal.;* **51**, **10**, 692.
Dalton K. (1973). *Proc. Roy. Soc. Med.;* **66**, 3 , 262–266.
Dalton K. (1975). *Headache;* **12**, **4**, 151–159.
Dalton K. (1976). *ibid;* **15**, **4**, 247–251.
Dalton K. (1982). Evidence submitted to FDA, Washington, Feb.
Frable M.A.S. (1962). *Arch. Otolaryngol;* **75**, 66.
Glass M. (1961). *Brit. Med. J.;* **1**, 1251.
Greene R. (1943). *Proc. Roy. Soc. Med.;* **36**, 306.
Greene R., Dalton K. (1953). *Brit. Med. J.;* **1**, 1007.
Hanley S.P. (1981). *Brit. J. Dis. Chest;* **75**, 306.
Haspels A.A. (1981) *Premenstrual Syndrome*, Ed. van Keep P. and Utian W.H., **6**, 81–92.
Hutfield D.C. (1961). *Brit. Med. J.;* **1**, 906.
Kerr G.D., Day J.B., Munday M.R., Brush M.G., Watson M., Taylor R.W. (1980). *Practitioner;* **224**, 852–855.
Ray A.M. (1961). *Brit. Med. J.;* **1**, 590.
Rees L. (1963). *J. Psychosom. Res.;* **7**, 191.
Smith S.L., Sauder C. (1969). *Psychosom. Med.;* **31**, **4**, 281–287.

Chapter 8

Benedek-Jaszmann L.J., Hearn-Sturtevant M.D. (1976). *Lancet;* **i**, 1985.
Dalton K. (1954). *Brit. Med. J.;* **2**, 1071.
Dalton K. (1957). *Proc. Roy. Soc. Med.;* **50**, **6**, 415.
Dalton K. (1964). *Premenstrual Syndrome*, William Heinemann Medical Books, London.
Dalton K. (1982). Evidence submitted to FDA, Washington, Feb.
Greene R., Dalton K. (1953). *Brit. Med. J.;* **1**, 1007.
Janiger O., Riffenburgh R., Kersch R. (1972). *Psychosomat.;* **13**, 226–235.
Kantero R.L., Widholm C. (1971). *Acta Obstet. Gynec. Scand. (Suppl.);* **14**, 7–18.

Kessel N., Coppen A. (1963). *Lancet;* **ii**, 61.
Lloyd T.S. (1963). *Virg. Med. Month;* **90**, 51.
Logan W.P.D., Cushion A.B. (1958). *Morbidity Statistics in Gen. Pract.;* **1**, (Gen.) London HMSO.
Pennington V.M. (1957). *J. Amer. Med. Ass.;* **164**, 638.

Chapter 9

Bäckström T. (1976). *Acta Neurol. Scand.;* **54**, 321–347.
Bäckström T. (1978). *Senologia;* **3**, 15–26.
Bäckström T. (1983). *Progesterone and Progestins,* Ed. Bardin C.W., Milgröm E., Mauvais-Jarvis P., Raven Press, New York, 203–217.
Bäckström T., Aakvaag A. (1981). *Psychoneuroendocrin;* **6**, 245–251.
Bäckström T. Cartensen H. (1974). *J. Ster. Biochem;* **5**, 257–260.
Bäckström T. Cartensen H. (1976). *ibid;* **7**, 469–471.
Benedek-Jaszmann L.J., Hearn-Sturtevant M.D. (1976). *Lancet;* **i**, 1095–1098.
Costa D.J., Bonnycastle D.D. (1952). *Arch. Int. Pharmacodyn;* **91**, 330–338.
Dalton M.E. (1981). *Postgrad. Med. J.;* **57**, 560–561.
Dalton M.E. (1984). *J. Ster. Biochem;* Jan.
Halbreich U., Ben-David M., Assael M., Bornstein R. (1976). *Lancet;* **ii**, 654.
Iqbal M.J., Johnston M. (1977). *J. Ster. Biochem.;* **8**, 977–985.
Jeske W., Klos J., Perkowncz J. and Stopinska U. (1980). *Materio Med. Polona;* 1–2, 42.
Merryman W., Boiman R., Barnes L. & Rothchild I. (1954). *J. Clin. Endocrin. Metab.;* **14**, 1567–1569.
Munday M. (1977). *Curr. Med. Res. Opin.;* **4**, Suppl 4, 16–22.
Munday M.R., Brush M.G., Taylor R.W. (1981). *Clin. Endocrin;* **14**, 1–9.
Reid R.L., Yen S.S.C. (1981). *Amer. J. Obstet. Gynec.;* **139**, 1, 85–104.
Süteri P.K., Fabrest F., Clemens L.E., Chang R.J., Gondos B., Stites D. (1977). *Ann. New York Acad. Sci.;* 384–397.
Speroff L., Glass R.H., Kase N.G. (1938). *Clinical Endocrinology and Infertility,* Williams and Wilkins, Baltimore/London.
Spiegel E., Wyeis H. (1945). *J. Lab. Clin. Med.;* **30**, 947–955.

Chapter 10

Allen W.M., Corner G.W. (1929). *Amer. J. Physiol.;* **88**, 340–346.
Allen W.M. (1974). *Gynec. Inv.;* **5**, 142–182.
Corner G.W., Allen W.M. (1929). *Amer. J. Physiol.;* **88**, 326–339.
Dalton K. (1964). *The Premenstrual Syndrome,* William Heinemann Medical Books, London.
Dalton K. (1968). *Brit. J. Psych.;* **516**, 114, 1377.
Dalton K. (1976). *ibid;* **129**, 438.
Dalton M.E. (1984). *J. Ster. Biochem.;* Jan.
Granger L.R., Roy S., Michell D. (1982). *Amer. J. Obstet. Gynec.;* **144**, **5**, 578–583.
Herbert A.L., Robboys I., MacDonald G.J., Scully R.E. (1974). *Amer. J. Obstet. Gynec.;* 607.
Jeffcoate, Sir N. (1975). *Principles of Gynaecology,* Butterworth, London.

Jenkins J.S. (1961). *Brit. Med. J.;* **4**, 861–863.
Johansson E.D.B. (1971). *Acta Endocrin;* **68**, 779–792.
Johansson E.D.B. (1971) *Amer. J. Obstet. Gynec.;* **110**, 4, 470.
Jones G.S. (1983). *Progesterone and Progestins,* Ed. Bardin C.W., Miligram E., and Mauvais-Jarvis P., Raven Press, New York.
Kerr G.D., Day J.B., Munday M.R., Brush M.G., Watson M., Taylor R.W. (1980). *Practitioner;* **103**, 390–402.
Landau R.L., Bergenstal D.M., Lugibihl K., Krischt M.E. (1955). *J. Clin. Endocrin.;* **15**, 1194.
Landau R.L., Lugibihl K., Bergenstal D.M., Dimick D.F. (1957). *J. Lab. Clin. Med.;* **50**, 613.
Loraine J.A., Beller E. (1971). *Hormonal Assays & Their Clinical Applications,* Livingston S., London.
Nillius S.J., Johansson E.D.B. (1971). *Amer. J. Obstet. Gynec.;* **110**, 4, 470.
Rothchild I. (1983). *Progesterone and Progestins,* Ed. Bardin C.W., Milgram E. and Mauvais-Jarvis P., Raven Press, New York, 231–245.
Speroff L., Glass R.H., Kase N.G. (1983). *Clinical Gynaecologic Endocrinology and Infertility,* 2nd Ed. Williams & Wilkins Co., Baltimore, US.
Thorne G.W., Engel L.L. (1938), *J. Exp. Med.;* **68**, 299.
Victor A., Weiner E., Johansson E.D.E (1977). *Acta Endocrin;* **86**, 430–436.
Wilkins L. (1960). *J. Amer. Med. Ass.;* **172**, 1028.

Chapter 11

Abraham G. (1981). *Current Problems Obstet. Gynec.;* **3**, 12, 539.
Benedek-Jaszmann L.J., Hearn-Sturtevant M.D. (1976). *Lancet;* **i**, 1095–1098.
Clare A.W. (1982). *J. Psychosomat. Obstet. Gynecol;* **1**, 22.
Ghose K.I., Cappen A. (1977). *Brit. Med. J.;* **1**, 148.
Graham J.J., Harding P.E., Wise P.H., Berriman H. (1978). *Med. J. Aust. Suppl.;* **3**; 18–20.
Horrobin D.F., Brush M.G. (1983). *Int. Symp. Premenstrual Tension & Dysmen.,*S. Carolina, Sept.
Keep van P., Utian W.H. (1981). *The Premenstrual Syndrome,* MTP Press Ltd., Lancaster, England.
O'Brien P.M.S., Craven D., Selby C., Symmonds E.M. (1979). *Brit. J. Obstet. Gynaec.;* **86**, 142–147.
O'Brien P.M.S., Selby C., Symmonds E.M. (1980). *Brit. Med. J.;* **1**, 1161–1163.
Radwanska E., Berger G.S., Hammond J. (1979). *Obstet. Gynec.;* **54**, 789–792.
Smith S.L. (1975). *Topics in Psychoendocrinology,* Ed. Sachar E.J., Grune & Stratton, New York.

Chapter 12

Dalton K. (1968). *Brit. J. Psych;* 114, 1377–1382.
Dalton K. (1976). *ibid;* 129, 438.
Dalton K. (1983). Evidence submitted to the FDA, Washington, Feb.
Herbert A.L., Robboys I., MacDonald G.J., Scully R.E. (1974). *Amer. J. Obstet. Gynec;* 607.
Johansson E.D.B. (1969). *Acta Endocrin.;* Copenhagen **61**, 607.

Johansson E.D.B. (1971). *Amer. J. Obstet. Gynec.;* **710, 4**, 470.
Lynch A., Mychalkiw W., Hutt S.J. (1978). *Early Human Devel.;* 2/4, 305–322.
Nillius S.J., Johansson E.D.B. (1971). *Amer. J. Obstet. Gynec.;* **710, 4**, 470.
Zussman J.U., Zussman P.P., Dalton K. (1975). *Soc. Research Child Devel.,* Denver.

Chapter 13

Dalton M.E. (1984). *J. Ster. Biochem.;* Jan.
Nillius S.J., Johansson E.D.B. (1971). *Amer. J. Obstet. Gynec.;* **710, 4**, 470.
Sampson G. (1979). *Brit. J. Psych.;* **135**, 209–211.
Smith S.L. (1975). *Topics in Endocrinology,* Ed. Sackar E.J., Raven Press, New York.

Chapter 14

Dalton K. (1962). *J. Obstet. Gynec.;* **69**, 3.
Dalton M.E. (1981). *Postgrad. Med. J.;* **57**, 560–561.
Nillius S.J., Johansson E.D.B. (1971). *Amer. J. Obstet. Gynec.;* **110, 4**, 470.
Van der Meer Y.G., Van Loenen A.C., Loendersloot E.W., Jaszmann L.J.B. (1982). *Pharm. Weekblad. Sci. Ed.;* **4**, 135–136.

Chapter 15

Dalton K. (1962). *J. Obstet. Gynaec. Brit. Comm.;* **69**, 3.
Dalton K. (1964). *The Premenstrual Syndrome,* William Heinemann Medical Books, London.
Nillius S.J., Johansson E.D.B. (1971). *Amer. J. Obstet. Gynec.;* **110, 4**, 470.
Nillius S.J., Johansson E.D.B. (1971). *Acta Endocrin.;* **1, 68,** 4, 17–20.

Chapter 17

Abraham G.E., Lubran M.M. (1981). *Amer. J. Clin. Nut.;* 2364–2366.
Abeaux-Fernet M., Loublie G. (1946). *Sem. Hop. Paris;* **22,** 1487.
Beaumont P.J.V., Richard D.H., Golder M.G. (1975). *Brit. J. Psychiat.;* **123**, 431–434.
Benedek-Jaszmann L.J., Hearn-Sturtevant M.D. (1976). *Lancet;* **i,** 1095–1098.
Clare A.W. (1982). *J. Psychosomat. Obstet. Gynec.;* **1**, 22–31.
Coppen A., Kessel N. (1963). *Brit. J. Psychiat.;* **109**, 711–721.
Dalton K. (1957). *Brit. Med. J.;* **2**, 378.
Dalton K. (1959). *ibid;* **2**, 1307.
Dalton K. (1962). *J. Obstet. Gynaec. Brit. Comm.;* **69**, 3.
Dalton K. (1968). *Brit. J. Psychiat.;* **516**, 114, 1377.
Dalton K. (1973). *Headache;* **12, 4**, 151.
Dalton K. (1976). *Brit. J. Psychiat.;* **129**, 438–442.
Day J.B. (1979). *Postgrad. Med. J.;* **109**, 711–712.
Elsner C.W., Buster J.E., Schindler R.A., Nissim S.A., Abraham G.E. (1980). *Obstet. Gynec.;* **56, 6**, 723–726.

Foresti G., Ferraro M., Reithaar P., Beerlanda C., Volpi M., Drago O., Cerutti R. (1981) *Psychother. Psychosom.*; **36**, 37–42.
Gray L.A. (1941). *Sth. Med. J.*; **34**, 1004.
Green R., Dalton K. (1953). *Brit. Med. J.*; **1**, 1007.
Haskett R.F., Steiner M., Osmun N., Carroll J.B. (1980). *Bio. Psychiat.*; **15**, 1, 121–139.
Janiger O., Riffenburgh R., Kersh R. (1972). *Psychosomat*; **13**, 226–235.
Kerr G.D., Day J.B., Munday M. Brush M.G., Watson M., Taylor R.W. (1980). *Practitioner*; **224**, 852–855.
Moos R.H. (1968). *Psychosom. Med.*; **30**, 853–867.
Moos R.H. (1969). *Amer. J. Obstet. Gynec.*; 390–402.
Oelkers W., Schöneshöfer M., Blümel A. (1974). *J. Clin. Endocrin. Metab.*; **39**, 882–883.
Osborn M. (1981). *J. Psysomat. Res.*; **138**, 339–405.
Puech A. (1942). *Montpellier Med.*; **21–2**, 118.
Radwanska E., Berger G.S., Hammond J. (1979). *Obstet. Gynec.*; **54**, 789–792.
Sampson G.A., Prescott P. (1981). *Brit. J. Psychiat.*; **138**, 339–405.
Singer K., Cheng R., Schou M. (1974). *Brit. J. Psychiat.*; **124**, 50–51.
Whitehead M.I., Townsend P.T., Gill D.K. (1980). *Brit. Med. J.*; **280**, 825–828.
Wood C., Jakubowicz D. (1980). *Brit. J. Obstet. Gynaec.*; **87**, 627–630.

Chapter 18

Dalton K. (1975). *Sports Medicine*, Ed. Williams J.G.P., Sperryn E., Arnold, London.

Chapter 19

Dalton K. (1969). *The Menstrual Cycle*, Penguin Books Ltd, London.
Fuch F. (1982). *Behaviour and the Menstrual Cycle*, Ed. Friedman, R., Marcel Dekker Inc., New York, **10**, 199–216.
Kessel N., Coppen A. (1963). *Lancet*; **ii**, 61.
Lennane K., Lennane R.J. (1973). *New Engl. J. Med.*; 288, 288.

Chapter 20

Allen W.M. (1974). *Gynec. Inv.*; **5**, 142–183.
Bennett F.O. (1939) *N.Z. Med. J.*; **38**, Obst. Gynaec. Sect. 11.
Dalton K. (1954). *Brit. Med. J.*; **2**, 1071.
Dalton K. (1955). *Medical World*; Dec. 1–4.
Dalton K. (1957). *Brit. Med. J.*; **2**, 378–381.
Dalton K. (1960). *Lancet*; **i**, 198–199.
Dalton K. (1962). *J. Obstet. Gynaec. Brit. Comm.*; **LXIX**, 3, 463–468.
Dalton K. (1968). *Brit. J. Psychiat.*; **114**, 1377–1382.
Dalton K. (1976). *ibid*; **129**, 438–442.
Dalton K. (1981). *Neuropharmacology*; **20**, 1267–1269.
Greenhill J.P., Freed S.C. (1940). *Endocrin.*; **26**, 529.

McMann W. (1938). *Va. Med. Mon.*; **65**, 676.
Marsden G.E. (1937),. *Brit. Med. J.*; **2**, 1221.
Oakley W. (1953). *ibid.*; **1**, 1413.
Paterson S. (1938–9). *Trans. Edin. Soc.*; **98**, 49.
Rothchild I. (1983). *Progesterone and Progestins,* Ed. Bardin C.W., Milgram E., Mauvais-Jarvis P., Raven Press, New York, 219–229.
Sammour M.B., El-Kabarity H., Khalifa A.S. (1975). *Acta Obstet. Gynaec. Scand.*; **54**, 195–202.

Chapter 21

Boyd, D.A. (1942). *Amer. J. Obstet. Gynec.*; 149–163.
Dalton K. (1971). *Brit. J. Psychiat.*; 118, 547.
Dalton K. (1971). *Proc. Roy. Soc., Med.*; **64**, **12**, 1249–1252.
Dalton K. (1980). *Depression After Childbirth,* Oxford University Press, Oxford.
Foundeur M., Fixsen C., Triebel W.A., White M.A. (1957). *Arch. Neurol. Psychiat.*; **77**, 503–512.
Hegarty A.B. (1955). *Brit. Med. J.*; **1**, 637.
Hoffman, F., v Lam L. (1948); *Zbl. Gynäk;* **70**, 1177.
Malleson J. (1963). *Brit. Med. J.*; **2**, 158.
Pitt B. (1968). *Brit. J. Psychiat.*; **114**, 1325–1335.
Pitt B. (1973). *ibid;* **122**, 431–443.
Ryle A. (1961). *J. Ment. Sci.*; **107**, 279–286.
Schmidt H.J. (1943). *J. Amer. Med. Ass.*; 190–192.
Soltau D.H.K., Taylor N.H. (1982). *Brit. Med. J.*; 284, 981.
Tod E.D.M. (1964). *Lancet;* ii, 264.
Yalom I.D., Lunde D.T., Moss R.H., Hamburg D.A. (1968). *Arch. Gen. Psychiat.*; **18**, 16.

Chapter 22

Bishop P.M.F., Richards N.A. (1952). *Brit. Med. J.*; 1, 244.
Bishop P.M.F., Richards N.A., Doll R. (1956). *Brit. Med. J.*; **2**, 130.
Csapa A., Pahanka O., Kaihola L.H. (1973). *Lancet;* ii, 1097.
Dalton K. (1969). *The Menstrual Cycle,* Penguin Books Ltd, London.
Johansson E.D.B. (1969). *Acta Endocrin.,* Copenh.; **61**, 607.
Jones S.G. (1973). *Obstet. Gynec.*; **26–34.**
Jones S.G. (1983). *Progesterone and Progestins,* Ed. Bardin C.W., Milgram E., Mauvais-Jarvis P., Raven Press, New York, 189–202.
Swyer G.I.M., Daley D. (1953). *Brit. Med. J.*; **1**, 1073.

Chapter 23

Bäckström T., Boyle H., Baird D.T. (1981). *Brit. J. Obstet. Gynecol.*; **88**, 530–536.
Barker M.G. (1968). *Brit. Med. J.*; **2**, 91.

Cooke I.D. (1976). *The Management of the Menopause and Post-Menopausal Years*, Ed. Campbell S., MTP Press Ltd, Lancaster, England, 49–62.
Dalton K. (1957). *Proc. Roy. Soc. Med.;* **50**, 6, 415.
Dalton K. (1964). *The Premenstrual Syndrome*, William Heinemann Medical Books, London 70–76.
Dalton K. (1969). *The Menstrual Cycle*, Penguin Books Ltd, London.
Denderstein L., Ryan M. (1982). *J. Psychosomat. Obstet. Gynec.;* **1–2**, 81–86.
Gray A.L. (1941). *South Med. J.;* **34**, 1004.
Greene R., Dalton K. (1953). *Brit. Med. J.;* **1**, 1007.
Lauritzen C. (1975). *Front Hormone Res.;* **3**, 21–31.
Richards, D.W. (1973). *Lancet;* **ii**, 430.
Studd J.W.W., Thom M.H., Paterson M.E.L., Wade-Evans J. (1980). *Menopause and Post Menopause*, MTP Press Ltd, Lancaster, 127–139.

Chapter 24

Dalton K. (1960a). *Brit. Med. J.;* **1**, 326–328.
Dalton K. (1960b). *ibid;* **2**, 1425–1426.
Dalton K. (1960c). *ibid;* **2**, 1647–1649.
Dalton K. (1961). *ibid;* **2**, 1752–1753.
Dalton K. (1964). *Proc. Roy. Soc. Med.;* **57**, 4, 262.
Dalton K. (1966). *ibid;* **59**, 10, 1014–1016.
Dalton K. (1968). *Lancet;* **ii**, 1386.
Dalton K. (1980). *ibid;* **ii**, 1070–1071.
Dalton K. (1982). *World Medicine;* 17th April.
D'Orban P.T., Dalton J. (1980). *Psychol. Med.;* **10**, 353–359.
McClinton M.K. (1971). *Nature;* **229**, 244, 5282.
Pierson W.R., Lockhard A. (1963). *Brit. Med. J.;* **1**, 796.
Taylor L., Dalton K. (1983). *California Western Law Review;* **19**, 2, 269–287.

Chapter 25

Dalton K. (1966). *Proc. Roy. Soc. Med.;* **59**, 10, 1014.
Dalton K. (1968). *Lancet;* **ii**, 1386.
Dalton K. (1969). *The Menstrual Cycle*, Penguin Books, London.
Dalton K. (1970). *Brit. Med. J.;* **2**, 27–28.
Dalton K. (1977). *J. Mat. Child Health;* 69–73.
Henderson M. (1978). Private communication.
McClinton M. (1971). *Nature;* **229**, **244**, 5282.
Tuch R. (1975). *Psychosomat. Med.;* **37**, 4, 388–394.

Original papers by
Dr Katharina Dalton

1953 'The premenstrual syndrome' (Joint authorship with Raymond Greene) *British Medical Journal*, vol i, p 1007.

1954 'Similarity of symptomatology of premenstrual syndrome and toxaemia of pregnancy and their response to progesterone' *British Medical Journal*, vol ii, p 1071. (Charles Oliver Hawthorne BMA Prize.)

1955 'Discussion on the premenstrual syndrome' *Proceedings of the Royal Society of Medicine* vol 48, No 5, pp 337–347.

1957 'The aftermath of hysterectomy and oopherectomy' *Proceedings of the Royal Society of Medicine*, vol 50, No 6, pp 415–418.

1957 'Toxaemia of pregnancy treated with progesterone during the symptomatic stage' *British Medical Journal*, vol ii, pp 378–381.

1959 'Menstruation and acute psychiatric illnesses' *British Medical Journal*, vol i 2, p 236.

1959 'Comparative trials of new oral progestogenic compounds in treatment of premenstrual syndrome' *British Medical Journal*, vol ii, pp 1307–1309.

1960 'Early symptoms of pre-eclamptic toxaemia' *Lancet*, pp 198–99.

1960 'Effects of menstruation on schoolgirls' weekly work' *British Medical Journal*, vol i, pp 326–328.

1960 'Menstruation and accidents' *British Medical Journal*, vol ii, pp 1425–1426.

1960 'Schoolgirls' behaviour and menstruation' *British Medical Journal*, vol ii, pp 1647–1649.

1961 'Menstruation and crime' *British Medical Journal*, vol ii, pp 1752–1753.

1962 'Controlled trials in the prophylactic value of progesterone in the treatment of pre-eclamptic toxaemia' *Journal of Obstetrics and Gynaecology of the British Commonwealth*, vol LXIX, No 3, pp 463–468.

1963 'The present position of progestational steroids in the treatment of premenstrual syndrome' *Medical Women's Federation journal*, pp 137–140.

1966 'The influence of mother's menstruation on her child' *Proceedings of the Royal Society of Medicine*, vol 59, No 10, pp 1014–1016. (Charles Oliver Hawthorne BMA Prize.)

1967 'Influence of menstruation on glaucoma' *British Journal of Ophthalmology* vol 51, No 10, pp 692–695. (Charles Oliver Hawthorne BMA Prize.)

1968 'Ante-natal progesterone and intelligence' *British Journal of Psychiatry* vol 114, pp 1377–1382.

1968 'Menstruation and examinations' *Lancet*, vol ii, pp 1386–1388.

1970 'Children's hospital admissions and mother's menstruation' *British Medical Journal* vol ii, pp 27–28.

1971 'Prospective study into puerperal depression' *British Journal of Psychiatry*, vol 118, No 547, pp 689–692.

1971 'Puerperal and premenstrual depression' *Proceedings of the Royal Society of Medicine*, vol 64, No 12, pp 1249–1252.

1973 'The general practitioner and research' *Practitioner*, vol 210, pp 784–788.

1973 'Progesterone suppositories and pessaries in the treatment of menstrual migraine' *Headache* vol 12, No 4, pp 151–159.

1974 'Migraine in general practice' *Journal of the Royal College of General Practitioners* vol 23, pp 97–106 (Migraine Trust Prize 1972).

1975 'The effect of progesterone on brain function' *Proceedings of the Acta Endocrin Congress*, Amsterdam.

1975 'Post-pubertal effects of prenatal administration of progesterone' *Society for Research in Child Development*. (Joint authorship Zussman J. and Zussman P.)

1975 'Food intake prior to a migraine attack – study of 2313 spontaneous attacks' *Headache*, vol 15, No 3, pp 188–193.

1976 'Migraine and oral contraceptives' *Headache*, vol 15, No 4, pp 247–251.

1976 'Prenatal progesterone and educational attainments' *British Journal of Psychiatry*, vol 129, pp 438–442. (Charles Oliver Hawthorne BMA Prize.)

1976 'A clinician's view of menopause' *Royal Society of Health Journal*, vol 92, No. 2, pp 75–77.

1976 'Bromocriptine and premenstrual syndrome' presented at the Symposium on Bromocriptine, Royal College of Physicians, London.

1978 'Menarcheal age in the disabled' *British Medical Journal*, **2**, p 475. Joint authorship with Maureen E. Dalton.

1979 'Intelligence and prenatal progesterone: A reappraisal' *Journal of the Royal Society of Medicine*, vol 72, pp 387–399.

1979 'Food intake before migraine attacks in children' *Journal of the Royal College of General Practitioners* No 29, pp 662–665. Joint authorship Michael J. T. Dalton.

1979 'Intelligence and prenatal progesterone' *Journal of the Royal Society of Medicine* vol 72, p 951.

1980 'Cyclical criminal acts in premenstrual syndrome' *Lancet*, ii, pp 1070–1071.

1981 'The effect of progesterone and progestogens on the fetus' *Neuropharmacology*, December.

1982 'The importance of diagnosing premenstrual syndrome' *Health Visitor*, vol 55, p 66. February 1982.

1982 'The legal implications of premenstrual syndrome' *World Medicine*, 17 April 1982.

1982 'What is this premenstrual syndrome?' *Journal of the Royal College General Practitioners*, December, pp 717–719.

1983 'Premenstrual syndrome: a new criminal defense?' *Calif. West. Law, Rev.* 19, 2, pp. 269–287. (Joint authorship with Laurence Taylor.)

Books by Dr Katharina Dalton

1964 *Premenstrual Syndrome* published by Wm. Heinemann Medical Books, London (translated into Spanish).

1969 *The Menstrual Cycle* published by Penguin Books, Harmondsworth, London and Pantheon Books, Random House, New York (translated into Spanish, Portuguese, French, Dutch, German, Swedish, Norwegian and Danish).

1975 *Women in Sports* (Chapter *Sports Medicine)*, Williams J.G.P., Sperryn P.N., E. Arnold, London.

1977 *Premenstrual Syndrome and Progesterone Therapy*, published by Wm. Heinemann Medical Books, London, and Year Book Medical Publishers Inc., Chicago.

1978 *Once a Month*, published by Fontana Paperbacks, London and Hunter House Inc., Pomana, USA (translated into Dutch and Indonesian).

1980 *Depression after Childbirth*, published by Oxford University Press, Oxford. (translated into Dutch, Japanese and German).

1982 *An Overview – Premenstrual Tension*, Chapter 11, *Menstruation and Behaviour*. Ed. R. Friedman, Marcel Dekker, New York.

Index